T0175484

INTEGRATED CARE

A Guide for Effective Implementation

INTEGRATED CARE

A Guide for Effective Implementation

Edited by

Lori E. Raney, M.D.

Gina B. Lasky, Ph.D., M.A.P.L.

Clare Scott, L.C.S.W.

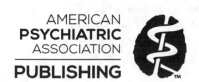

AMERICAN
PSYCHIATRIC
ASSOCIATION
PUBLISHING

Note: The authors have worked to ensure that all information in this book is accurate at the time of publication and consistent with general psychiatric and medical standards, and that information concerning drug dosages, schedules, and routes of administration is accurate at the time of publication and consistent with standards set by the U.S. Food and Drug Administration and the general medical community. As medical research and practice continue to advance, however, therapeutic standards may change. Moreover, specific situations may require a specific therapeutic response not included in this book. For these reasons and because human and mechanical errors sometimes occur, we recommend that readers follow the advice of physicians directly involved in their care or the care of a member of their family.

Books published by American Psychiatric Association Publishing represent the findings, conclusions, and views of the individual authors and do not necessarily represent the policies and opinions of American Psychiatric Association Publishing or the American Psychiatric Association.

If you wish to buy 50 or more copies of the same title, please go to www.appi.org/specialdiscounts for more information.

Copyright © 2017 American Psychiatric Association Publishing

ALL RIGHTS RESERVED

21 20 19 18 17   5 4 3 2 1

American Psychiatric Association Publishing
1000 Wilson Boulevard
Arlington, VA 22209-3901
www.appi.org

Library of Congress Cataloging-in-Publication Data
Names: Raney, Lori E., 1960– editor. | Lasky, Gina, 1974– editor. | Scott, Clare, 1953– editor. | American Psychiatric Association, issuing body.
Title: Integrated care : a guide for effective implementation / edited by Lori E. Raney, Gina Lasky, Clare Scott.
Other titles: Integrated care (Raney)
Description: Arlington, Virginia : American Psychiatric Association Publishing, [2017] | Includes bibliographical references and index.
Identifiers: LCCN 2017009983 (print) | LCCN 2017011458 (ebook) | ISBN 9781615370542 (alk. paper) | ISBN 9781615371334 (ebook)
Subjects: | MESH: Delivery of Health Care, Integrated | Primary Health Care | Mental Health Services
Classification: LCC RA418 (print) | LCC RA418 (ebook) | NLM W 84.1 | DDC 362.1—dc23
LC record available at https://lccn.loc.gov/2017009983

British Library Cataloguing in Publication Data
A CIP record is available from the British Library.

Contents

Part I
A Design for Success

Part II
The Provider Role: Changing Practice

Part III
Operational Considerations

Contributors

Chris Keenan, M.D., M.P.H.
Clinic Medical Director, Clinica Family Health, Lafayette, Colorado

John Kern, M.D.
Clinical Professor of Psychiatry and Behavioral Sciences, University of Washington School of Medicine, Seattle, Washington

Gina B. Lasky, Ph.D., M.A.P.L.
Senior Consultant, Health Management Associates, Denver, Colorado

Ron Manderscheid, Ph.D.
Executive Director, National Association of County Behavioral Health and Developmental Disability Directors, Washington, D.C.; Adjunct Professor, Department of Mental Health, Bloomberg School of Public Health, Johns Hopkins University, Baltimore, Maryland

Kristan McIntosh, L.M.S.W.
Senior Consultant, Health Management Associates, New York, New York

Consuelo Elizabeth Mendez-Shannon, M.S.W., Ph.D.
Project Director for Hispanic/Latinx Affairs, Office of the Vice President for Diversity and Inclusion, Iowa State University, Ames, Iowa

Gaylee Morgan, M.P.P.
Vice President, Health Management Associates, Chicago, Illinois

Lori E. Raney, M.D.
Principal, Health Management Associates, Dolores, Colorado

Julianna Reece, M.D., M.B.A., M.P.H.
Family Medicine Physician, Durango, Colorado

Kristen Roessler, M.D., FAAP
Study Physician, Center for American Indian Health, Johns Hopkins Bloomberg School of Public Health; Staff Pediatrician, Cortez Integrated Health Center, Cortez, Colorado

Clare Scott, L.C.S.W.
Consultant, Collaborative Care Consulting, Lafayette, Colorado

Carolyn Shepherd, M.D.
Principal, Leibig-Shepherd, LLC, Boulder, Colorado

Jack Todd Wahrenberger, M.D., M.P.H.
Medical Director for Primary Care, Pittsburgh Mercy Family Health Center, Pittsburgh, Pennsylvania

Rob Werner, B.A.
Senior Consultant, Health Management Associates, Chicago, Illinois

DISCLOSURES OF INTEREST

All contributors to this book have reported no competing interests during the year preceding manuscript submission.

Foreword

In 1948, the World Health Organization defined health as "a state of complete physical, mental and social well-being and not merely the absence of disease or infirmity."[1] Effective integration of primary care and behavioral health care can take us a long way toward realizing this goal. Three decades of research have demonstrated that effective collaboration between primary care and mental health professionals can improve health outcomes. Over the past decade, this research has been summarized in a number of meta-analyses and books, and today there is widespread acceptance that effectively integrated care can improve access to care and health outcomes for individuals and populations of patients. Despite compelling research evidence, however, most patients do not have access to integrated care, and when organizations attempt to integrate behavioral health care, they do not always use approaches with documented effectiveness. Barriers to the widespread implementation of evidence-based programs include payment and regulatory barriers, lack of a workforce trained in effective collaboration, and cultural differences between the worlds of primary care and behavioral health care. For decades, primary care providers and mental health specialists have worked in relative isolation from each other, but today we live in a time where we are learning that effective "sharing" of problems, information, and resources can help us accomplish more than when we are engaged in "parallel play." Information technology and a willingness to share have brought us innovative companies such as Uber and Airbnb. The same spirit can help us make effective use of mental health specialists who are a limited resource in all but a handful of affluent communities in the United States.

---

[1]Preamble to the Constitution of the World Health Organization as adopted by the International Health Conference, New York, 19–22 June 1946; signed on 22 July 1946 by the representatives of 61 States (Official Records of the World Health Organization, no. 2, p. 100; World Health Organization 1948) and entered into force on 7 April 1948.

In this book, editors Lori E. Raney, M.D., Gina B. Lasky, Ph.D., M.A.P.L., and Clare Scott, L.C.S.W., have collected more than a decade's worth of practice experience on how to integrate behavioral health and primary care and how to build effective collaborative care teams. For those of us who are convinced that integrated care is the way forward, it is this kind of information that we need in order to change our practices, to build interdisciplinary care teams that enjoy working together, and to improve care for the patient populations we serve. The lessons shared in this book can help us anticipate and navigate many of the barriers to implementing effective integrated care, and I hope they will encourage us to share our own experiences with the growing community of patients, providers, health care organizations, and payers who are pursing the goal of integrated behavioral health care.

Jürgen Unützer, M.D., M.P.H., M.A.
Professor and Chair, Psychiatry and Behavioral Sciences,
University of Washington, Seattle, Washington

Introduction

The logic and benefits of bringing behavioral health (defined in this book as mental health and substance use disorders) and somatic medicine (care that is not typically considered behavioral health) together in an integrated care structure is being accepted by medical practices and introduced into specialty behavioral health centers throughout the United States. The advantages of integrated care from a clinical perspective are better detection of illness, improvement in overall health outcomes, and a better patient care experience, including reduced suffering. From an administrative perspective, it provides a foundation for responding to policy and finance changes that are happening in an unprecedented fashion and include an emphasis on return on investment and a move to value-based payment.

However, the actual implementation of this concept is complex and can be overwhelming. The good news is that there is an emerging framework of core principles, implementation research, and practice-based experience to serve as a guide. This information is useful in both traditional integration of behavioral health into general medical settings (often primary care) or integration of general medical care into specialty mental health or substance use treatment settings. Administrators, clinicians, policy makers, payers, and others need guidance in determining what effective implementation looks like. With that in mind, we designed this book to offer a three-part examination of key components of any implementation strategy and, along with our contributing authors, include essential elements for success. The chapter authors were selected for their direct clinical experience in various integrated environments, their leadership in ushering through these initiatives, and/or their deep knowledge of payment and policy barriers.

Integrated care for the purposes of this book is a nonspecific term that refers to a variety of approaches to provide physical and behavioral health care simultaneously, regardless of the location of practice. It assumes there is a care team practicing in a systematic way to provide an array of mental health, substance use, or physical health services in a typically nontraditional location in order to provide whole person care for a given population.

There are two typical approaches to integrating behavioral health and primary care with various modifications and a blending of the models practiced in different locations:

- The **Primary Care Behavioral Health model** has developed since the mid-1990s into an approach with extensive practice experience in providing immediate access to behavioral health providers for a variety of acute stressors and behavioral health conditions. This model also supports primary care providers in managing medical conditions where there is a need for behavioral intervention. The research on this model is limited by an absence of controlled trials, but findings have demonstrated evidence of primary care provider and patient satisfaction.
- The **Collaborative Care Model (CoCM)** is a specific type of integrated care with an extensive evidence base developed over the past two decades. With over 80 positive randomized controlled trials across numerous physical locations, diagnoses, ethnic groups, and payer populations, it is a model of integrated care that has demonstrated consistent outcomes and cost savings. It is therefore prudent to use this rich reservoir of data and mine it not only for its well-demonstrated effectiveness, but also for a set of fundamental unifying principles, implementation processes, and key features of team interactions that contributed to this success. For this reason the editors of this book chose to focus on the research accumulated from trials of the CoCM including emerging implementation effectiveness research.

As outlined below, this book is organized into three parts and includes an appendix of performance and outcome measures:

- **Part I—A Design for Success** lays the groundwork for effective integrated care by exploring key features of success across three chapters. Chapter 1, "Elements of Effective Design and Implementation," describes the evidence base for the CoCM. The chapter presents the Core Principles of Effective Integrated Care, derived by an expert consensus panel, and the details of key implementation research projects. The author then introduces a set of care model factors that coincided with better outcomes. These care model factors become the backbone for many of the remaining chapters in the book. Chapter 2, "Organizational Leadership and Culture Change," covers the vital need for strong leadership in any effort to integrate primary care and behavioral health and ways to successfully reach this goal. Chapter 3, "Team Development and Culture," tackles the myriad issues that surface when the cultures of somatic medicine and behavioral health begin to merge. The author offers valuable approaches to successful team formation and culture shift.

- **Part II—The Provider Role: Changing Practice** covers the key clinical players on the care team, including the behavioral health provider (psychologist, social worker, therapist, or behavioral care manager), the primary care provider (physician, nurse practitioner, or physician assistant), and the psychiatric consultant (psychiatrist, psychiatric nurse practitioner, or physician assistant). Chapter 4, "Behavioral Health Provider Essentials," is written by two seasoned behavioral health providers who share their research and practical experience in working in these roles. Chapter 5, "The Primary Care Provider," is written by an experienced and talented group of primary care providers and may be the most comprehensive coverage of integrated primary and behavioral health care currently available. Chapter 6, "The Psychiatric Consultant," defines the role of the psychiatric consultant and describes in detail the force multiplier effect of indirect consultation, which is the key to extending scarce psychiatric expertise across larger populations in need.
- **Part III—Operational Considerations** discusses practical operational aspects of integrated care. Chapter 7, "Policy and Regulatory Environment," examines the interplay between policy and practice transformation in relationship to integration. Chapter 8, "Financing Integrated Care," examines the complex financing landscape and the impacts of integrating physical and behavioral health care.
- The **Appendix: Performance and Outcome Measures for Integrated Care** is provided for evaluating effectiveness in clinical, financial, and operational aspects of integrating care.

Acknowledgments

All the authors of this book have our deepest appreciation for their hard work, thoughtful approach, and rich expertise that make this book a success. We also thank the American Psychiatric Association Publishing leadership and staff for conceiving of a multidisciplinary book and for guiding us through the process.

LORI RANEY, M.D.

I wish to start with thanking my coeditors Gina B. Lasky, Ph.D., M.A.P.L., and Clare Scott, L.C.S.W., for the wonderful opportunities we have had to work together and hone our thinking about effective implementation strategies. I also extend my gratitude to Jürgen Unützer, M.D., M.P.H., M.A., Anna Ratzliff, M.D., and John Kern, M.D., who have continued our work to better train and prepare psychiatrists and other team members to work in this field. The American Psychiatric Association staff, including Kristin Kroeger, Chief of Policy, Programs, and Partnerships, have been very instrumental in this effort and allowed us to get this information to many more psychiatrists and others with their hard work and dedication through the Transforming Clinical Practice Initiative. I also want to thank my colleague Nancy Kamp, whose work on effective implementation inspired the outline for some parts of this book. My husband, Don Raney, has continued his unwavering support for this work, and I thank him for his helpful late-night edits and ideas.

GINA B. LASKY, PH.D., M.A.P.L.

I would like to thank Margaret Kaems, L.C.S.W., and Carolyn Shepherd, M.D., for sharing their rich experience and expertise on the day-to-day work of leadership and team development. Their time and energy improved these chapters and brought the material to life. I'd also like to thank Steve Scoggin, M.Div., Psy.D., L.P.C., and Sharon Raggio, L.P.C., L.M.F.T., M.B.A., for their early review and recommendations that enhanced the discussion of culture change.

I am in deep gratitude for my team members Lori E. Raney, M.D., and Clare Scott, L.C.S.W., who led me to collaborative care. They have shared countless hours of expertise and knowledge, provided enduring vision for the future of the approach, and inspired my commitment to improving organizational implementation of integrated care. They both have been true team members in my life personally and professionally.

I would like to thank my parents, who instilled a passion for value-based leadership, and my six siblings, who taught me from an early age the hard work and incredible reward of working as a team. Last, I would like to thank my husband, David, for his endless support and humor through all my adventures!

CLARE SCOTT, L.C.S.W.

This work would not have been possible without the foresight of Barbara Ryan, Ph.D., Pete Liebig, and Carolyn Shepherd, M.D., and their efforts to initiate and sustain a Collaborative Integration Program Partnership between a community mental health and a community health clinic. Thank you to Janet Rasmussen and Emily Vellano for their continued leadership with the model. Our success was dependent on medical leads Chris Keenan, M.D., M.P.H., and Jeff Almony, M.D., and none of our work could have happened without a dedicated group of behavioral health professionals, including Lynn Scheidenhelm, Michael Dow, Jennifer Peck, Marja Dansie, Kestrel Hanson, Susana Gonzalez, and Fern Hemmer, who trusted and assisted me in developing a brand-new way of working. Thanks to Jim Mellblom for creating a simple diagram to illustrate a very complex role, and to my husband, Michael Scott, for his continued support.

Part I

A Design for Success

CHAPTER 1

Elements of Effective Design and Implementation

Lori E. Raney, M.D.

SETTING THE STAGE: THE NEED FOR EFFECTIVE IMPLEMENTATION

This is a seminal moment in the evolution of the clinical integration of behavioral health and somatic medicine. As an established innovation, it is increasingly apparent that this approach is important to the success of the Triple Aim in health care (Berwick et al. 2008. Therefore, there is an urgency to do it correctly and to ground practice implementation in the research on effectiveness. Only then can we ensure that integration meets these goals of improved clinical outcomes, containment of cost, and improvement in the patient experience of care. Incorporating research on implementation is crucial to the long-term success of current health care reform efforts such as patient-centered medical homes (PCMHs), accountable care organizations (ACOs), and other developing approaches to health care system transformation. Only with purposeful alignment of successful strategies can these system shifts reach these core tenets, and it is these effective models that will allow value-based payment structures to be meaningful.

As seen by the numerous approaches to integrating primary care and behavioral health (defined in this book as both mental health and substance use disorders), the field is evolving, and consistent evidence is emerging about both tangible and intangible factors that can lead to success. We are learning that integration occurs best within the bounds of an evidence-based framework that is emerging through implementation research and that this frame-

3

work can lead to better outcomes and cost containment. Without these core components, the research points to a lack of clinical progress and ultimately a failure to deliver on defined outcomes. At risk is frustration for payers and health systems when seemingly commonsense methods (such as simple co-location of behavioral health staff in a primary care clinic) fail to reach desired outcomes. Systems of care lose credibility when models do not work, subsequently resulting in loss of funding. If the failure is one of implementation rather than the actual research components of an innovation, then the whole system loses a valuable advancement. Even more distressing is the long-term possibility that the "failed attempt" at integrated care will be viewed as a "failed idea," and an incredible opportunity will be lost. In a growing field, there is the need to understand factors that do not work and why, while providing solutions to overcome what are common errors in design and implementation.

Real innovation requires a strategic and thoughtful approach with skills in areas such as leadership, culture change, and selecting the right people for the tasks required. It requires understanding the nuances of integration and the research regarding what makes it work, a commitment to the process that goes beyond half measures or convenience, and the humility to realize personal and professional characteristics that can be barriers in an environment of merging cultures. Transformative change requires real change.

Models

Collaborative Care Model

Extensive empirical literature supports the Collaborative Care Model (CoCM) as an effective method of integrating primary care and behavioral health (see the section "Evidence Base for Collaborative Care" later in this chapter). This model incorporates behavioral health providers (BHPs or behavioral care managers) and psychiatric consultants (psychiatrists, psychiatric nurse practitioners, or physician assistants with psychiatric certification) into primary care teams and then follows a systematic approach of measurement-based care and intervention for patients not improving as expected. The CoCM is a population-guided approach that tracks all patients in the defined group in a data management tool called a *registry*, allowing accountability to the system for outcomes for a designated subset. It is unique in its use of psychiatric consultation for curbside consultation and caseload review, with very limited direct patient care. This indirect approach allows an extension of limited psychiatric expertise to larger populations in need, increasing the reach of this limited resource by an estimated order of magnitude. One limitation of this approach is that it is often diagnosis specific (e.g., focusing on depression or anxiety), and there may not be immediate accessibility of the BHP for a "warm handoff" from the primary care provider (PCP) or to help with other behavioral health issues in the clinic.

Primary Care Behavioral Health or Behavioral Health Consultant Model

The Primary Care Behavioral Health (PCBH) approach to integrated care places a behavioral health consultant on the primary care team to provide immediate interventions for acute life stressors, crises, mental health and substance use disorders, stress-related physical symptoms, and ineffective patterns of health care utilization, and to provide referral to higher-level-of-specialty behavioral health services as needed. PCPs appreciate the immediate availability of the behavioral health consultant to address issues and help keep the clinic flow on track. But this approach rarely includes a psychiatric consultant as part of the team for curbside consultation or to help with patients who are not improving as expected, although co-located psychiatric services may be available through traditional referral. In addition, systematic repeat measurement of progress tracked in a registry is typically not part of the approach, which makes it difficult to demonstrate outcomes.

Blended Model

An ideal approach might be to use a "blended" method that combines the PCBH model and the CoCM. The blended model is appropriate when there are enough behavioral health resources to address patients with episodic stressors in an immediate fashion, as well as a subset of this population with identified, specific behavioral health conditions that can receive the more rigorous collaborative care approach. In the CoCM, treatment response is systematically measured, results are tracked in a registry, and a process is in place to initiate a change in treatment for patients who are not progressing as expected. Additionally, regular caseload reviews with a psychiatric consultant are part of the strategy to routinely evaluate outcomes and change course as needed. This blended approach is utilized in many clinics already, and as long as there are adequate resources this approach may be preferable.

With a focus in this chapter on the research of implementation from multiple trials of the CoCM, it is time to think beyond specific "models" per se and focus attention on what is necessary for any approach to change outcomes. An "all hands on deck" attitude (Unützer 2016) allows using a blended approach., which could incorporate 1) components of the PCBH model for addressing issues such as acute stressors and health behavior change (Robinson and Reiter 2016) and 2) elements of the CoCM, when a defined diagnosis such as depression or anxiety will be treated and tracked until targeted outcomes are reached. Embracing a "perennial philosophy" (Mauksch and Fogarty 2016) in the field where there is agreement on what makes integration successful can help bridge professional guilds and disciplines and allow a braiding of approaches to provide effective and timely care.

A Framework for Action

The multiple clinical trial replications resulting in the robust evidence base for the CoCM have led to a distillation of features into a set of Core Principles of Effective Integrated Care, and emerging implementation research is revealing key process-of-care tasks and the distinctive elements (or "secret sauce") that bind these principles into a cohesive structure. While implementation research continues, the goal is to use the existing knowledge to develop an effective system of care that can successfully treat mild to moderate mental illness, the "sweet spot" of intervention in the primary care setting. Intentionally being rigorous does not mean being rigid or fanatical; thus, attention to the needs and resources of a specific clinic setting is valid and important. Weaving together the Core Principles and implementation research findings allows for flexibility in the design of methods. For example, employing practical steps initially, with adoption of additional necessary evidence-based components when resources are available, can be a real-world approach to getting started without being overly strict and delaying any implementation progress. In the end, the goal is to encourage a higher aspirational vision of truly effective integrated care, and this book is designed to assist in creating approaches that PCMHs, ACOs, payers, and others can count on to deliver the real promise of effective and cost-effective whole person care.

Core performance measures that go beyond screening rates and provider or patient satisfaction will be a desired approach as behavioral health specialists deliver the outcomes and cost containment required (see the appendix, "Performance and Outcome Measures for Integrated Care"). For example, Medicaid ACO regulations have added National Quality Forum standard 710 (i.e., depression remission at 12 months) as a performance measure, which will require a robust approach to treatment (see www.cms.gov/medicare/ medicare-fee-for-service-payment/sharedsavingsprogram/downloads/ ry2015-narrative-specifications.pdf). In addition, the Center for Medicare and Medicaid Services has released billing codes tied closely to the CoCM that will require understanding and performing key tasks in this approach in order to receive reimbursement (see www.cms.gov/Newsroom/MediaReleaseData base/Fact-sheets/2016-Fact-sheets-items/2016-07-07-2.html and Chapter 8, "Financing Integrated Care").

EVIDENCE BASE FOR COLLABORATIVE CARE

The CoCM was conceptualized by Wayne Katon, M.D., at the University of Washington (Katon et al. 1995) and over time has evolved into a model with an extensive evidence base. The core structure of the approach is modeled on the Chronic Care Model (Wagner et al. 1996) that employs a process of health care delivery redesign with a proactive team-based approach. This structure was used to inform the first large-scale study of collaborative care called the Improving Mood—Promoting Access to Collaborative Treatment (IMPACT) intervention for the treatment of depression in older adults (Unützer et al. 2002). Subsequently, over 80 randomized controlled trials have been conducted using the structure of the IMPACT model (now collectively known as the CoCM) and have demonstrated effectiveness across multiple treatment settings, populations, diagnoses (Table 1–1), and payer groups (Archer et al. 2012; Garrity 2016; Gilbody et al. 2006; Thota et al. 2012). In addition, when depression and common medical conditions such as hypertension and diabetes are treated concurrently in studies such as TEAMcare (Katon et al. 2010) and Collaborative Care Model for Patients with Depression and Diabetes and/or Cardiovascular Disease (Rossom et al. 2016), significant improvements are seen in both the behavioral health and other medical conditions. The evidence base also extends to the child and adolescent population with good results (Asarnow et al. 2015).

TABLE 1–1. Evidence base for the Collaborative Care Model by diagnosis

Evidence base established	Emerging evidence
• Depression	• Substance use disorders
• Depression and chronic medical conditions	• Attention-deficit/hyperactivity disorder
• Anxiety	• Bipolar disorder
• Posttraumatic stress disorder	
• Chronic pain	
• Dementia	

An analysis of total health care costs 4 years following the conclusion of the IMPACT trial demonstrated a return on investment of $6 for every $1 spent implementing the model (Unützer et al. 2008) and an estimate that widespread implementation could save as much as $28–$46 billion (Melek et al. 2014). A pay-for-performance approach has shown the effect of withholding payment until key process and outcome measures are met, further demonstrating the ability to use the structure of the model to incentivize the team to reach robust outcomes (Unützer et al. 2012).

CORE PRINCIPLES OF
EFFECTIVE COLLABORATIVE CARE

A set of Core Principles of Effective Collaborative Care, distilled from multiple clinical trials of the CoCM and established during an Expert Consensus Summit at the University of Washington in 2011 (https://aims.uw.edu/ collaborative-care/principles-collaborative-care), provides key features that can serve as a guide to designing an effective approach. The mnemonic TEMP-A can be useful for remembering these principles, described further in Table 1–2:

- **T**eam based and patient centered
- **E**vidence based
- **M**easurement based
- **P**opulation based
- **A**ccountable

DEFINING THE POPULATION
FOR INTERVENTION

The process starts by defining the population of patients to receive the collaborative care intervention so that the right problem is being addressed. Data analytics (e.g., electronic medical record extracts, claims data) are the preferred way to identify the population, rather than a "hunch" that certain conditions are more prevalent than others, although some diagnoses, such as depression, may be mandatory for inclusion. Data analytics also provide a baseline against which quality measures can be benchmarked. The type of intervention employed is dependent on the availability of local resources to treat the behavioral health issues encountered, which should be considered as the population is determined. Although universal screening for specific conditions may be optimal, lack of sufficient resources to perform the necessary follow-up could hamper attaining successful outcomes, so selection of a subset of the population may be warranted. In some locations, such as federally qualified health centers and other federal facilities, mandatory depression screening with the Patient Health Questionnaire–2 (PHQ-2; Kroenke et al. 2003) is required at defined intervals whether or not adequate resources

TABLE 1–2. Core Principles of Effective Integrated Care: TEMP-A

Team based and patient centered	PCPs and BHPs collaborate effectively on care teams using shared care plans that incorporate patient goals.
Evidence based	Patients are offered treatments such as brief psychosocial interventions and medications for which there is credible research evidence to support their efficacy in treating the target condition.
Measurement based	Each patient's care plan clearly articulates personal goals and clinical outcomes that are routinely measured. Treatments are adjusted if patients are not improving as expected.
Population based	The care team shares a defined group of patients tracked in a registry to make sure no one "falls through the cracks." Practices track and reach out to patients who are not engaging or progressing as expected, and psychiatric consultants provide caseload-focused consultation on all patients who are not improving, not just ad hoc advice on select patients.
Accountable	Providers are accountable and reimbursed for quality care and outcomes.

Note. PCPs = primary care provider; BHPs = behavioral health providers.
Source. Adapted from Raney L: *Integrated Care: Working at the Interface of Primary Care and Behavioral Health.* Arlington, VA, American Psychiatric Publishing, 2015; and adapted from https://aims.uw.edu/collaborative-care/principles-collaborative-care. Used with permission.

are available for follow-up. Many clinics use the PHQ-2 with an algorithm to complete the full Patient Health Questionnaire–9 (PHQ-9) if the score on the PHQ-2 is positive. Although this may seem to be easier, it causes difficulties in long-term follow-up for patients with depression for the reasons mentioned in Box 1–1.

Box 1–1.   A Word of Caution: Using the PHQ-2 versus the PHQ-9 for initial screening

There are several issues to consider when deciding which tools to use for screening purposes. For several reasons the PHQ-9 (Kroenke et al. 2001), although longer, may be the best option initially instead of the PHQ-2.

- It is important to understand that the scores on the PHQ-2 and PHQ-9 are not interchangeable and therefore should not be compared to each other over time; each screening tool requires separate entry mechanisms.
- The PHQ-2 is often given verbally by someone placing a patient in the exam room, and the results may vary based on how the question is asked (and received) by the patient. Often the PHQ-2 is asked as a "yes" or "no" question instead of using the scoring in the actual tool, potentially picking up more false negatives.
- Patients may disclose more on self-reported measures.
- The PHQ-9 picks up a lot of distress, including many physical and other symptoms that can help identify other disorders in addition to depression (such as anxiety or substance use disorders).
- The PHQ-9 takes 3–5 minutes to complete and is not overly burdensome.
- The PHQ-9 picks up mild depression (score 5–9) and allows an opportunity for self-management interventions and prevention of more severe symptoms.
- Once a person has been treated for depression, it is better to use the PHQ-9 (and not revert back to "screening" with the PHQ-2) so that relapse can be detected in the mild range.

Data might reveal a high rate of women with postpartum depression or a school-based health center with an increase in referrals following a school-wide depression screening initiative. Patients with one or more chronic conditions (such as diabetes, hypertension, and asthma) historically have high rates of behavioral health conditions, and if a clinic's data confirm this is true for their site, then this group could become the targeted population for intervention. One helpful approach is gathering data that demonstrates certain trends: for example, 1) the rate of behavioral health conditions in a primary care setting (including pediatrics and obstetrics/gynecology); 2) the rate of behavioral health diagnoses in patients with one or more/two or more chronic conditions (see Table 1–3 as an example); 3) psychiatric disorder diagnoses in the top 10% of frequent utilizers of the emergency department; or 4) behavioral health diagnoses in patients with 30-day readmissions following a hospital discharge.

MEASUREMENT-BASED CARE

Measurement-based care (MBC) is defined as the systematic use of validated measurement tools to adjust treatment to reach desired outcomes. In behavioral health, MBC has lagged behind that of other medical specialties, making it difficult for psychiatrists and other BHPs to demonstrate value in the services they provide. More recently, enhanced by experience gained in the success of the CoCM and other studies, closer attention has been paid to the potential of utilizing this process to improve outcomes in behavioral health. In a study of psychiatrists, Guo and colleagues (2015) demonstrated how, even with the most highly trained specialists, MBC dramatically improved both treatment response, time to response, and improvement in rates of remission.

This approach is at the heart of the success of the CoCM, which at its core is an elegant model of delivering MBC. In 2015, Patrick Kennedy and a team at the Kennedy Forum announced a National Call for Measurement-Based Care in the Delivery of Behavioral Health Services, complete with three issues briefs covering integrated care, a scientific review of the evidence base, and key features of MBC, as well as a supplement, "Core Set of Outcome Measures for Behavioral Health Across Service Settings" (https://www.thekennedyforum.org/resources). A follow-up to this effort was the publication of an article in a peer-reviewed journal by the Kennedy Forum team lead by Fortney and colleagues (2016), describing key concepts gleaned from an extensive review of the existing literature on MBC in behavioral health.

Effective approaches to MBC summarized from the literature review include frequent administration of the measurement tools and timely feedback of results to the provider. Ineffective approaches include one-time screening, infrequent assessment, and giving the results to providers outside the current clinical situation (Fortney et al. 2016). Although MBC is specifically designed to impact decision making at the individual patient level, the authors

TABLE 1–3. Example of clinic data gathered: behavioral health diagnoses in patients with chronic medical conditions

	Patients in primary care with disorder	Patients with comorbid behavioral health disorder	Behavioral health diagnosis
Diabetes	26%	36%	Depression
Hypertension	22%	28%	Depression and anxiety equal
Asthma	18%	42%	Anxiety
Arthritis	15%	39%	Depression
Chronic pain	15%	62%	Depression and opiate dependence

also describe potential secondary gains, including the use of aggregate data for professional development and quality improvement, as well as informing payers about outcomes necessary to demonstrate value—similar to results reported for other medical conditions (Fortney et al. 2016).

STEPPED CARE APPROACH

The core tasks of the collaborative care process follow a stepped care pattern (Von Korff and Tiemens 2000) and are based on three assumptions:

• Different people need different levels of care for the same problem.
• Monitoring outcomes helps determine the right level.
• Moving along the stepped care continuum from lower to higher levels can improve outcomes and contain costs.

Starting with self-management techniques and watchful waiting for sub-syndromal symptoms and progressing up the stepped care ladder, interventions can be undertaken by the PCP alone, the PCP in collaboration with the BHP, or the PCP and BHP with the psychiatric consultant. Referral to specialty behavioral health resources outside of the primary care clinic, including short-term and longer-term therapies or psychiatric inpatient treatment, represent the highest levels of care and resource utilization. Depending on need, patients may skip levels if more intensive resources are clearly what is needed at a given point in time.

The outcome of this resource-managing process on a population level is to effectively treat the majority of mild to moderate behavioral health conditions in the primary care setting while preserving specialty behavioral health services, including direct psychiatric evaluation for those who need this higher level of care. This approach can help overcome the typical scenario of limited access to specialty behavioral health services and more severely ill patients cycling though emergency departments, inpatient psychiatric facilities, inpatient medical/surgical units, and intensive care units because of an inability to access timely treatment. Another benefit is that by effectively treating conditions while they are in the mild to moderate range, there is an opportunity to prevent more severe conditions from occurring.

PROCESS OF CARE

The key tasks associated with care include detection of illness (including screening), assessment for confirmation of diagnosis, patient engagement through frequent follow-up, initiating treatment, promoting adherence, tracking and adjusting care as needed through caseload review and psychiatric consultation, care coordination, referral (if needed), promoting patient self-management, and quality improvement. Each task is handled in a specified manner to provide the best chance of good outcomes.

Screening Tools

Once the patient population is defined, the next step is identification of behavioral health conditions through the use of patient (or family) report and select screening tools. Patients present differently in the primary care setting. Chief complaints such as unexplained pelvic pain, stomach cramps, headaches, fatigue, and palpitations may mask an underlying behavioral health condition. Behavioral health screening tools are analogous to a set of "vital signs" that help detect previously unrecognized conditions, resulting in a set of comprehensive vital signs when combined with the typical array performed when starting a medical visit.

Table 1–4 lists commonly used screening tools. It is important to remember these tools are for identifying symptoms and are not the sole instruments in diagnosing specific conditions. Discussing the findings with the patient to further explore the situation is a necessary prerequisite to establishing a definitive diagnosis, and these tools do not replace good clinical judgment.

Some PCPs are reluctant to do screening for behavioral health conditions because of concerns that it will lead to additional problems to address that they do not have the time or clinical skills necessary to provide effective treatment, and that it will extended the length of appointments and cause delays in an already hectic schedule. However, without these tools PCPs may avoid inquiring about a patient's emotional state even when this could clearly be compromising their ability to adequately treat a patient's other medical conditions. This issue is a significant contributor to PCP reluctance to participate in a collaborative treatment approach and must be addressed up front to reassure them that this is a team-based model and support is reliably there specifically to manage behavioral health diagnoses (see Chapter 5, "The Primary Care Provider").

Treatment of the Identified Condition(s)

Treatment starts with the crucial element of engaging patients in care and proceeds to diagnostic clarification. If an acute stressor is identified that does not meet the level of a psychiatric diagnosis, or a health behavior intervention is needed and a blended model is being used, a brief onetime session with no plan for follow-up could take place at this juncture. This stopgap measure can be a valuable tool in addressing behavioral health issues before they progress to a diagnosable problem, adding an element of prevention to the primary care

TABLE 1–4. Commonly used screening tools in primary care settings

Mood disorders	Anxiety disorders	Psychotic disorders	Substance use disorders	Cognitive disorders
PHQ-9: depression (score >9 or positive on question 9)	GAD-7: anxiety, GAD (score >7) PTSD–PC: PTSD	Brief Psychiatric Rating Scale Positive and Negative Syndrome Scale	AUDIT: alcohol use (score >7 for women and score >8 for men)	Mini-Mental State Examination Mini-Cog
MDQ: bipolar disorders CIDI: bipolar disorders			Number of heavy drinking days Drinking below risky drinking limits.[a]	Montreal Cognitive Assessment
			CAGE Questionnaire: alcohol use DAST: drug use	

[a]No more than 7 drinks a week or 3 at a time in women and anyone over the age of 65 and no more than 14 drinks a week or more than 4 drinks at a time for men under the age of 65.

Note. AUDIT = Alcohol Use Disorders Identification Test; CAGE = Cutdown, Angry, Guilty, Eye opener, a screen for alcohol use; CIDI = Composite International Diagnostic Interview for Bipolar Disorder; DAST = Drug Abuse Screening Test; GAD-7 = Generalized Anxiety Disorder 7-item scale; MDQ = Mood Disorder Questionnaire; PHQ-9 = Patient Health Questionnaire–9; PTSD–PC = Posttraumatic Stress Disorder–Primary Care.

Source. Adapted from Raney L: *Integrated Care: Working at the Interface of Primary Care and Behavioral Health.* Arlington, VA, American Psychiatric Publishing, 2015. Copyright © 2015 American Psychiatric Publishing. Used with permission.

setting. Alternately, patients with more severe mental illnesses may present to primary care, where having a BHP there who understands the psychopathology and can assist in a referral to specialty behavioral health care is invaluable. If disorders such as depression, anxiety, or substance use are identified through the screening and assessment procedures of the BHP and PCP, then the process of initiating and providing collaborative care treatment would follow (for specific approaches by the care team members, see Chapter 4, "Behavioral Health Provider Essentials"; Chapter 5, "The Primary Care Provider"; and Chapter 6, "The Psychiatric Consultant"). This level of collaborative care usually includes proactive and persistent outreach, frequent symptom measurement with validated tools, brief behavioral interventions (e.g., motivational interviewing, behavioral activation; see Chapter 4 for complete list), promoting adherence to medications and other interventions, psychiatric consultation, education, and self-management strategies. While Screening, Brief Intervention, and Referral to Treatment (Bernstein et al. 2007) is not a model of integrated care, it is evident this process of care fits nicely into the core functions already occurring in the CoCM.

Using a Registry to Track Response and Caseload Review

A crucial step in effective integrated care is the tracking of patient-specific results in a data management tool called a registry. This process begins with entering the initial measurement score (such as the baseline PHQ-9 for depression or GAD-7 [Generalized Anxiety Disorder 7-item scale] for anxiety) and other clinical data that are relevant to care tracking. Registries provide a method to prevent patients from getting "lost to follow-up" and to notify the team of tasks that are needed (such as repeat measurement), providing a mechanism for outreach. This tracking of response continues with regular measurement until remission, maximum attainable improvement, and/or referral to higher care is achieved. Data from the registry is used to identify patients who are not improving as expected so that treatment adjustments can be initiated during the regularly scheduled caseload reviews with the psychiatric consultant. All team members and administrators utilize the registry for various tasks. Chapter 4 demonstrates how the BHP uses the registry; Chapters 5 and 6, respectively, show how the PCP and psychiatric consultant use the data that are collected. Table 1–5 demonstrates the types of data that could be entered into a registry created from a simple Excel spreadsheet, and an online resource for a registry to use in integrated clinics can be found here: http://aims.uw.edu/resource-library/patient-tracking-spreadsheet-example-data.

TABLE 1–5. Example of a registry and psychiatric consultant recommendations

Patient ID	Diagnosis	Initial visit[a]	Last visit[a]	BL PHQ-9	Last PHQ-9	% change	BL GAD-7	Last GAD-7	% change	Psychiatric consultation[a]	Recommendations and comments
101	MDD	1/12/16	4/30/16	16	10	↓38	1	1	NA	3/15/16	Behavioral activation, increase sertraline to 100 mg
102	MDD, PTSD, chronic pain	2/2/16	5/12/16	18	22	↑18	12	11	↓8	3/31/16 4/15/16	Referral to chronic pain group, agreed to start duloxetine
103	Social phobia	2/10/16	4/14/16	1	1	NA	18	22	↑18	4/15/16	Discontinue bupropion, start citalopram 10 mg and increase in 1 week to 20 mg
104	MDD	9/12/15	4/14/16	17	3	↓32	0	0	NA	1/3/16	Relapse prevention plan and discontinue registry tracking

[a]Date of visit or consultation, by month/day/year.

Note. BL=baseline; GAD-7=Generalized Anxiety Disorder 7-item scale; ID=identification; MDD=major depressive disorder; PHQ-9=Patient Health Questionnaire–9; PTSD=posttraumatic stress disorder.

Using Aggregate Data to Improve Performance

Aggregate data from the registry can be used to track performance measures for the defined population and to inform quality improvement projects. This important step can be used for continuous quality improvement and combined with processes such as the Plan-Do-Study-Act cycle (see www.ihi.org/resources/pages/tools/plandostudyactworksheet.aspx for more information). Data-driven initiatives can lead to rapid improvements in the collaborative care treatment process. Decisions regarding changes in the workflow, adding staff, or initiating new treatment strategies are best informed by using a data-driven approach, ensuring a team addresses the right problem and that the treatment approach is working to deliver on predetermined outcomes. Box 1–2 provides an example of performance improvement.

**Box 1–2.   Example of Performance Improvement:
Using aggregate data from a registry**

Aggregate data from five clinic registries in a health care system revealed better depression outcomes reflected in a more rapid time to 50% improvement in PHQ-9 scores in four of the clinics. One clinic had significantly different results, showing fewer patients reaching the planned target. The team looked at multiple factors that could be contributing to this finding, including demographic variables, severity of behavioral and physical health disorders, caseload size, number of patient contacts by the BHP, and time to psychiatric consultation. The variable discovered in the data analysis was time to psychiatric consultation for patients who were not improving. The one clinic with worse results only had resources for a psychiatric consultant to review the registry once a month while the other four had more frequent reviews. A quality improvement project was initiated and a leadership decision was made to provide financial resources to support additional psychiatric time to increase the monthly registry reviews to weekly in this clinic to see if the results would improve over a 6-month period. Repeat analysis 6 months later showed this clinic with additional resources had not only caught up but had surpassed the other four in achieving outcomes.

IMPLEMENTATION RESEARCH

Factors Associated With Successful Implementation

Even with this set of Core Principles (see Table 1 2) to guide the process, trials have demonstrated uneven outcomes, and resulted in consideration that other factors may be influencing the results (Bauer et al. 2011; Whitebird et al. 2014). Implementation research is in its infancy but is beginning to reveal key additional factors in care processes and operational strategies that contribute to success or failure and define the distinctive elements that bind the Core Principles together. Whitebird and colleagues (2014) performed extensive field interviews with clinical and administrative staff providing collaborative care in the Depression Initiative Across Minnesota: Offering a New Direction trial (Pietruszewski 2010) and ranked a list of nine key factors important to effective implementation and, subsequently, better outcomes. Additional trends were noted, further divided into factors that contributed to patient engagement and achieving remission (Whitebird et al. 2014). Table 1–6 contains the nine factors ranked from most to least influential. Two subsets of these factors related to effectiveness were chosen for further scrutiny, and demonstrated patient activation was strongly correlated with strong leadership support and the presence of a PCP "champion." In patients reaching remission, the presence of an engaged psychiatrist and the availability of financial support were crucial to an effective outcome. Subsequent chapters in this book will provide a more in-depth description of each of these core variables.

Adhering to Specific Tasks to Achieve Outcomes

One way to approach the implementation research for the CoCM is to take the Core Principles and identify the key process-of-care tasks associated with those principles. These tasks can then be compared with outcomes to see if the assumptions are associated (Table 1–7).

Using the list in Table 1–7, one study of depressed adults (Bao et al. 2016) looked at the two key process-of-care tasks, which included one or more BHP contacts within 4 weeks of initiation of treatment and at least one psychiatric consultation between weeks 8 and 10 for patients who were not improving by week 8. Fidelity to both processes was associated with a greater likelihood of achieving improvement in depression treatment with the BHP contact measure also resulting in a shorter time to improvement. This finding demonstrates the importance of the BHP quickly engaging patients in care to form a relationship that allows treatment to begin (see more on BHP engagement techniques in Chapter 4). In addition, if a psychiatric consulta-

TABLE 1–6. Ranking of factors important to effective implementation

Rank	Factor	Description
1	Operating costs of DIAMOND not seen as a barrier	This factor is specific to the DIAMOND trial itself. Some sites could not afford to implement the additional services while others could.
2	Engaged psychiatrist	The psychiatrist is responsive to the care team and intervenes with patients who are not improving.
3	PCP "buy-in"	Providers actively support the use of the model and refer patients to the collaborative care program.
4	Strong care manager	The right person is hired for this job and performs the duties well.
5	Warm handoff	Patients are referred face-to-face from the PCP to the BHP instead of a remote introduction.
6	Strong top leadership support	Leaders in the organization support and provide resources for the project.
7	Strong PCP "champion"	At least one PCP in the clinic works to promote the model among peers and others.
8	Care manager role well defined and implemented	The job responsibilities of the care manager are clear and not confused with case management or other duties. Adequate time, space to work, and support are provided.
9	Care manager on-site and accessible	Care manager is visible in the clinic and readily available to staff and patients.

Note. BHP=behavioral health provider; DIAMOND=Depression Initiative Across Minnesota, Offering a New Direction; PCP=primary care provider.
Source. Adapted from Whitebird et al. 2014.

TABLE 1–7. Core components and key tasks of the Collaborative Care Model

Core component and task	Operational definition of task
Patient identification and diagnosis	
Diagnose behavioral health problems and related conditions.	≥1 working diagnosis for common behavioral health conditions checked during episode.
Use valid measurement tools to assess and document baseline severity.	≥1 measures completed at baseline, for example, the Patient Health Questionnaire–9 (PHQ-9) to assess depression severity.
Engagement in integrated care program	
Initiate patient tracking in population-based registry.	Patient has ≥1 follow-up contact with the care manager within 4 weeks of initial contact.
Systematic follow-up, treatment adjustment, and relapse prevention	
Use population-based registry systematically to follow all patients.	No period(s) of ≥60 days between enrollment and discharge in which no contact occurs.
Monitor treatments response at each contact with valid outcome measures.	Patient has ≥1 measures based on valid instruments (e.g., PHQ-9 for depression) recorded at each follow-up.
Identify patients who are not improving to plan for medication adjustment.	If not improving, patient has had medication dosage adjustment, switching, or augmentation within 90 days since initial contact.
Create and support relapse prevention plan when patients are substantially improved.	Patient who has achieved improvement during episode receives a relapse prevention plan as documented in the registry.

TABLE 1–7. Core components and key tasks of the Collaborative Care Model *(continued)*

Core component and task	Operational definition of task
Systematic case review and consultation	
Conduct regular psychiatric caseload review for patients who are not improving.	Patient not improving within 8 weeks of initial contact receives ≥1 psychiatric evaluations as documented in registry.

Source. Adapted from Bao Y, Druss BG, Jung HY, et al: Unpacking Collaborative Care for Depression: Examining Two Essential Tasks for Implementation. *Psychiatric Services* 67(4):418–424, 2016. Copyright © 2016 American Psychiatric Association. Used with permission.

tion occurred between weeks 8 and 12 for patients who were not improving by week 8, there was a greater likelihood of improvement by week 24. Furthermore, in the COMPASS trial (Rossom et al. 2016) infrequent caseload reviews in 1 clinic resulted in the lowest depression response and remission scores of all 18 clinics. Timely caseload review provides consultation on the more difficult patients, allowing more psychiatric expertise to be provided to those in need to improve outcomes.

An unpublished study (Bennett et al. 2016) of 20,000 adults evaluated four individual patient markers of improvement and the fidelity to the associated care tasks in the collaborative care treatment process. The authors discovered that completion of these tasks led to an increase in the likelihood of response to treatment for depression. These four tasks were 1) initiating patient tracking in a population-based registry, 2) using the registry to systematically follow up on all patients, 3) monitoring treatment response at each contact with valid outcome measures, and 4) monitoring medication use and treatment side effects/complications (Bennett et al. 2016).

Teamwork and Leadership Contributions to Effective Implementation

Chapter 2, "Organizational Leadership and Culture Change" and Chapter 3, "Team Development and Culture," will address the significance of strong leadership support and team functioning, which are important contributions to the secret sauce of effective implementation. In the Whitebird et al. (2014) study, the staff noted key leadership qualities that included the following: feeling supported; leaders showing up for team meetings, reviewing reports and data, and giving feedback to the treatment team; and the staff's comfort level with discussing challenging situations or asking for help from their leaders (N. Jaeckels Kamp, personal communication, June 3, 2015). Without this support the implementers will struggle to carry out processes that lead to a high-functioning system of care.

PERFORMANCE MEASUREMENT

It is important to have a system to track key performance measures in order to report outcomes in multiple domains including process, outcome, utilization, and satisfaction measures. These measures inform on the clinical level any need to adjust treatment, such as the changes for a particular population being served or modification necessary due to the outcomes that are achieved. For administrators and payers, both clinical and financial outcomes can be vital in deciding whether or not to pay for integrated care and, if so, what measures of accountability will be required of a health system to receive funding. These elements (i.e., clinical and financial outcomes, measures of accountability) have already proved to be important in both Medicaid funding of collaborative care in some states and the development of new codes to pay for nonbillable services associated with the CoCM (see Chapter 8). Although performance measures for integrated care still need some fine-tuning, the appendix at the end of this book, "Performance and Outcome Measures for Integrated Care," provides current thinking on key performance measures that can be utilized now to demonstrate accountability for the care provided. The performance measures in the appendix have been derived from many of the key elements of effective implementation that have been previously discussed in this chapter and will be further elucidated throughout the remaining chapters of this book.

FRONTIERS IN IMPLEMENTATION RESEARCH

Task Sharing

Seventy-seven percent of the counties in the United States have a severe shortage of BHPs (Thomas et al. 2009), and globally the dearth of these trained professionals prevents addressing many of the world's pressing needs (Morris et al. 2013). However, many paraprofessionals can serve effectively in some roles of the BHP in a task-shifting or shared fashion (see also Chapter 4), separating out those tasks that do not require a higher level of clinical expertise (and licensure) and saving the limited availability of the expert clinicians for those duties needing more advanced skills. From *promotoras* to community health workers, AmeriCorps volunteers to community-based organizations such as senior citizens centers, an untapped paraprofessional workforce has the potential to demonstrate their ability to participate in the delivery of evidence-based collaborative care (Hoeft and Unützer 2015). One example of this concept is the Archstone Foundation's project with older adults (see http://aims.uw.edu/care-partners-bridging-families-clinics-and-communities-advance-late-life-depression-care), where community partner organizations staffed with paraprofessionals are part of the treatment team, providing interventions in the community to complement the work of the primary care–based staff. An evaluation of staffing patterns in one trial of collaborative care for mild to moderate depression demonstrated no differences in outcomes between the sites that were staffed with registered nurses and those staffed with certified medical assistants or licensed practical nurses (Pietruszewski et al. 2015). These paraprofessional providers were trained to deliver a specific depression education protocol in this study, an important and necessary step when using unlicensed staff who have not had the professional training that would be associated with a degree. Licensed staff should be available for a more severely ill population or those with other diagnoses such as substance use disorders. This exploration of staffing alternatives is a growing area of research, as health care systems struggle with finding a sufficient number of affordable providers to deliver effective care.

Using Technology in Integrated Settings

Although there is extensive evidence of the benefits of collaborative care and a knowledge of core components that make it successful, in many locations there are not enough psychiatric providers or BHPs to perform the essential duties. However, a range of opportunities using various forms of technology are available to fill some of the gaps, moving along a continuum from practice extenders such as patient-guided apps and online therapy services, to building PCP capacity to treat mild to moderate behavioral health conditions, to virtual patient visits using telemedicine technology. Many of these approaches are currently used as stand-alone models but have the potential to be used in combination. In addition, they may have the potential for synergy with the essential tasks of collaborative care and, conversely, collaborative care principles could improve the approach of some of these technologies. As discussed in this chapter, the success of collaborative care works by utilizing several key processes to ensure that measurement-based, treat-to-target care is being provided. This includes some tasks that could be assisted through the use of technology approaches described in Table 1–8.

Combining Technologies

The opportunity to use these technology solutions in combination are numerous. For instance, in the CoCM, telepsychiatry is already a part of the process for many sites, which may see 5%–10% of patients who are not improving through use of this approach. Telepsychiatry could be further combined with eConsult for the curbside consultations and even a Psych Med ECHO for education and complex case discussions. A patient-facing app could send repeat PHQ-9s to care managers and encourage patient self-care with reminders of activation goals. In a system using eConsult or Psychiatry ECHO, telepsychiatry could be employed for further evaluation of the more difficult presentations. A Psych Med ECHO could use eConsult for the PCPs to connect with the hub specialists between sessions.

While these technologies are currently within reach, it is imperative that we continue the research into the efficacy and return on investment of these

TABLE 1–8. Roles of technology in collaborative care

Technology	Features and functions
Practice extenders	
Web and mobile apps to provide resources for patients to better manage their conditions	Apps and voice and text messaging for self-management of symptoms, education, remote monitoring, repeat symptom measurement (such as the PHQ-9); saves staff time with follow-up calls, can help patients engage in their care plan, and provides reminders of goals such as those used in behavioral activation, as well as computerized psychotherapy
Building the capacity for primary care providers to treat behavioral health conditions	
Clinical decision support	Built into the electronic health record, provides information in the form of algorithms ("smart sets"), prescription information, etc., at the point of care to drive decision making and enhance learning opportunities
Telementoring and collaborative learning	Utilizes a specialist hub and multiple primary care spokes for didactic, consultative, and case-based learning; see Project ECHO (Extension of Community Healthcare Outcomes; http://echo.unm.edu)
Electronic consultation ("eConsult")	Timely access for primary care-to-specialist consultation with an online consultation platform, asynchronous communication with embedded educational component
Other consultative communication	Includes programs such as the National Network of Child Psychiatry Access Programs (see www.nncpap.org), which offer telephonic consultation, some telepsychiatry, and additional services such as remote care coordination

TABLE 1–8. Roles of technology in collaborative care *(continued)*

Technology	Features and functions
Building the capacity for primary care providers to treat behavioral health conditions (*continued*)	
Consultation telehub	All-in-one service to provide the core features of collaborative care remotely, including curbside consultation, registry review, telepsychiatry, and behavioral care management (Fortney et al. 2013), for sites that have low provider/patient volumes, limited access to behavioral health resources, or the desire to outsource behavioral health care
Virtual visits with psychiatric providers	
Telepsychiatry	Direct evaluation of a patient at an originating site by a psychiatric provider at a distant site via teleconferencing, provides services in difficult-to-reach areas, and helps with the geographic maldistribution of psychiatric providers; can involve some "teleteaming" services beyond direct evaluation; direct-to-consumer evaluations are a growing area of practice and also are used for teletherapy

approaches. Obtaining funding resources for these solutions, most of which do not include a billable face-to-face visit, will continue to be challenging in a fee-for-service rather than value-based payment environment. Legal and data privacy issues as well as keeping up to date with technology advances all need to be continually addressed in this rapidly evolving environment. Proper vetting and implementation of new technologies for behavioral health will be important.

Box 1–3 provides a case study of a health care system that integrated and adapted some of these telemedicine elements.

**Box 1–3.   Case Study: Using Technology to Provide
Integrated Care: Carolinas HealthCare System**

In 2013, Carolinas HealthCare System (CHS; one of the nation's largest not-for-profit systems in the country, with 40 hospitals and 900 care locations serving over 2 million patients a year) had a goal: To fully integrate behavioral health into its 200 primary care offices. We knew early on that we would use the CoCM as the inspiration for our model and also knew that we would have to innovate in some way to scale across such a large system in a timely way. CHS was already investing in telehealth with programs like tele-stroke and tele-ICU so we decided to "go virtual" with collaborative care in an initial pilot of 10 clinics. We deconstructed the BHP role and reconstructed it into a virtual team designed around each of the functions of that position using professional and paraprofessional staff according to the need. Most of the team, which has grown to 20, is located at workstations in a telehealth "bunker," but others work from remote locations, clearly an advantage of virtual care.

Now, when a patient presents to his or her PCP with a behavioral health need, that PCP can connect immediately with our team and have the patient assessed in real time by video. The array of services provided includes drug-dosing algorithms and consultation to the PCP, callback protocols for the patient with coaching and reassessments, and online tools such as myStrength and Beating the Blues. The PCP remains the treating physician prescribing all medications and ordering any additional testing as needed. In just 2 years, our Behavioral Health Integration (BHI) team has served over 5,000 patients now in 50 primary care practices. Our first 6 months of data (which is pre/post and not controlled) shows statistically significant decreases in PHQ-9 and GAD-7 scores, and hemoglobin A_{1c}, LDL, and total cholesterol levels; this data suggests encouraging trends toward decreased utilization of inpatient services, particularly on the medical side (along with a slight increase in outpatient utilization). In addition to these promising findings, there has been clear (and emphatic) satisfaction expressed by the PCPs using the service and a list of practices in our system wanting it as soon as possible. The approach has also attracted national attention, particularly given that we are tracking outcomes using a lean infrastructure, which is easier to scale, in a health care market that is ever more focused on value and cost. The team has also gained the reputation within our system as one of the most vibrant and enthusiastic teams to be a part of.

—*John Santopietro, M.D., Behavioral Health Service Line Director, Carolinas HealthCare System, North Carolina (personal communication, August 5, 2016)*

A RECIPE FOR SUCCESS

The current formula for success in delivering effective integrated care is derived from a combination of fidelity to the Core Principles of Effective Collaborative Care, adhering to certain key process-of-care tasks, and a unique mix of factors related to the selection and interactions of the team members. Table 1–9 provides a list of key features that organizations need to consider if they want to design outcome-changing and cost-effective health care delivery systems. One approach may be to start with currently available components and then build on the additional features as resources become available to complete the system. However, absence of key components can lead to a less than desirable final product. In the meantime, we can be guided by what we know works and what does not.

THE CONTINUUM OF COLLABORATIVE SERVICES AND CYCLE OF PATIENTS WITHIN THIS SYSTEM OF CARE

In the not-too-distant future there could be a health care system that has the capacity to address both physical and behavioral health conditions across a continuum of services that functions in a seamless fashion and has enough flexibility to adequately address the needs of a population, regardless of local resource restrictions. This ideal system is within reach if health care reform leads to alternative payment models to allow for creativity and expansion of evidence-based and practice-tested models of integrated care delivery. This system would entail the redesign of both primary care and specialty behavioral health services to provide care across a continuum of services that allows effective treatment to occur in the less resource-intensive setting of primary care. However, if needed, patients could step up to the level of care provided in the specialty behavioral health system for an episode of care, with the plan for the majority of patients to return to the primary care end of the continuum. The exception to this would be that some patients with serious mental illnesses will continue to need the resources and team-based

TABLE 1–9. Summary of the key ingredients of effective collaborative care

Core principles	Key process-of-care tasks	Team-centered qualities
Team based and patient centered	Having one or more contacts with patients in the first month	Strong leadership support
Evidence based	Tracking with a registry	Primary care provider buy-in and champions
Measurement-based treatment to target	Identifying patients who are not improving and adjusting treatment with caseload review by a psychiatric consultant	Engaged psychiatric consultant
Population based	Monitoring treatment response at each contact with a valid measurement tool	Well-defined and implemented role of the care manager (behavioral health provider)

approach, including primary care services, provided in specialty behavioral health. This continuum (see Figure 1–1) is explained in detail below.

Social Determinants of Health

The health of an individual and a population rests on the fabric of the social determinants of health, which is often a major contributor to many illnesses. This wider set of forces includes access to education, economic opportunities, social supports, and environmental conditions (as shown in the outer ring of Figure 1–1), and these forces contribute significantly to the success or lack of success in maintaining health. The fifth social determinant is access to the health care system.

Primary Care

Primary care practices in this new configuration will have the resources they need to manage mild to moderate behavioral health conditions effectively in a variety of ways, including on-site services, telehealth options, telementoring and capacity-building arrangements such as Psych Project ECHO, electronic consultation such as eConsult and other services, and the use of

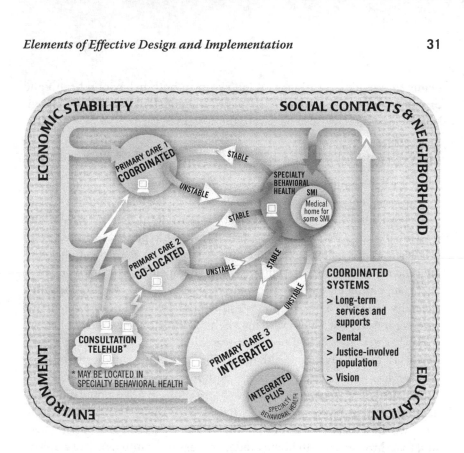

FIGURE 1–1. The continuum of collaborative services and cycle of patients within this system.

Note. SMI = patients with serious mental illness.
Copyright © Lori E. Raney, M.D.

consultation telehubs (see the section "Consultation Telehub" later in this chapter) that can remotely transport a team to their location. These practices will implement stepped care to efficiently use resources that provide effective treatment. Registries and psychiatric consultation will be used to adjust treatment for patients who are not improving, including referrals to higher levels of care if warranted. Acutely unstable patients can be quickly accommodated by a specialty behavioral health system that is reserved for those patients most in need. Primary care practices will help facilitate this availability through readily accepting patients back from specialty behavioral health care with behavioral health support when patients' conditions have stabilized and patients can be maintained safely within a primary care environment (such as is currently done with diabetes, cardiac disease, and other chronic health conditions). Connections to criminal justice and populations in need of long-term services and support will be facilitated by care teams to provide transitions and follow-up in both behavioral health and primary care settings. Adapting systems to adequately address oral and vision health issues will also be part of the system of care.

Specialty Behavioral Health

Specialty behavioral health services will be provided in an episodic manner for those patients who need a higher level of care. Once a course of treatment has been completed (e.g., dialectical behavioral therapy, alcohol use treatment, inpatient psychiatric admission), stable patients will return to primary care for follow-up and ongoing treatment (e.g., medication refills, ongoing measurement of symptoms, brief therapeutic interventions), freeing up appointments without an extensive waiting periods for new incoming specialty referrals. The exception to this approach will be those patients with serious mental illness who may benefit most from care management and other evidence-based practices provided in the specialty behavioral health site serving as their health home. These patients will receive primary care services in the setting that is best equipped for long-term recovery and health, as well as targeting the reduction in mortality in a population with demonstrated health disparities. A vital piece of the health home environment will be a focus on community and other population integration to ensure that through a health home model, there is no maintenance of a system of separate or segregated care for individuals with serious mental illness.

Consultation Telehub

Some primary care sites may use the services of a remote telehub to provide some or all of the behavioral health care that cannot be provided locally because of workforce or resource issues. Patients at these sites will have access to real-time direct care and specialty consultation as needed through a menu of services along the stepped care continuum of care. These services could include a patient referral to a paraprofessional in the hub for self-management and educational services, an "e-handoff" in the primary care setting by tablet to a BHP in the hub for diagnostic clarification and intervention, curbside consultations between the psychiatric consultant and the primary care–based team, evidence-based psychotherapy such as cognitive-behavioral therapy with a licensed therapist in the hub and a patient from his or her home or office by secure videoconferencing, weekly caseload reviews between a BHP at the primary care site and a psychiatric consultant in the hub, or direct evaluation through the use of telepsychiatry by the psychiatric consultant of select patients who are not improving. In addition, a specialist hub as demonstrated in a model like Project ECHO (noted earlier in the section

"Using Technology in Integrated Settings," see http://echo.unm.edu) could provide education through a case-based learning format to several remote spoke clinics (Arora et al. 2011). These consultation telehubs are being tested (Fortney et al. 2013), and several have already been developed around the United States. The Massachusetts Child Psychiatry Access Program, piloted in 2003 and implemented statewide in 2004, is an example of a successful system providing child psychiatric consultation, education, and direct care from an academic setting to distant pediatric primary care offices (see www.mcpap.com/Provider/McPAPservice.aspx).

CONCLUSION

Implementing effective integrated care is a complex process that requires attention to many important details. Much of the implementation of key processes has been derived from extensive clinical experiences and empirical research. If implemented with fidelity, these crucial components have demonstrated results that clinicians, payers, policy makers, and patients can rely on to move health care redesign forward. Delivery system restructuring and technology can address the need for more and better care with models that not only improve the care delivered but also address workforce shortages by using these new models. This restructuring could be accomplished by ensuring that patients with less debilitating behavioral health conditions receive care in primary care settings, while specialty behavioral health is reserved for patients with a greater burden of illness. Resources and funding as well as an openness to new technologies and attention to measurement-based care will be crucial to success.

REFERENCES

Archer J, Bower P, Gilbody S, et al: Collaborative care for depression and anxiety problems. Cochrane Database Syst Rev 10:CD006525, 2012 23076925

Arora S, Thornton K, Murata G, et al: Outcomes of treatment for hepatitis C virus infection by primary care providers. N Engl J Med 364(23):2199–2207, 2011 21631316

Asarnow JR, Rozenman M, Wiblin J, et al: Integrated medical-behavioral care compared with usual primary care for child and adolescent behavioral health: a meta-analysis. JAMA Pediatr 169(10):929–937, 2015 26259143

Bao Y, Druss BG, Jung HY, et al: Unpacking collaborative care for depression: examining two essential tasks for implementation. Psychiatr Serv 67(4):418–424, 2016 26567934

Bauer AM, Azzone V, Goldman HH, et al: Implementation of collaborative depression management at community-based primary care clinics: an evaluation. Psychiatr Serv 62(9):1047–1053, 2011 21885583

Bennett I, Mao J, Chan Y, et al: Association of pragmatic fidelity measures to collaborative care tasks with response to treatment of adult depression in primary care. Abstract accepted for NIMH Conference on Mental Health Services Research: Harnessing Science to Strengthen the Public Health Impact, Bethesda, MD, August 1–2, 2016

Bernstein E, Bernstein J, Feldman J, et al: An evidence based alcohol screening, brief intervention and referral to treatment (SBIRT) curriculum for emergency department (ED) providers improves skills and utilization. Subst Abus 28(4):79–92, 2007 18077305

Berwick DM, Nolan TW, Whittington J: The triple aim: care, health, and cost. Health Aff (Millwood) 27(3):759–769, 2008 18474969

Fortney JC, Pyne JM, Mouden SB, et al: Practice-based versus telemedicine-based collaborative care for depression in rural federally qualified health centers: a pragmatic randomized comparative effectiveness trial. Am J Psychiatry 170(4):414–425, 2013 23429924

Fortney JC, Unutzer J, Wrenn G, et al: A tipping point for measurement-based care. Psychiatr Serv 68(2):179–188, 2016 27582237

Garrity M: Evolving models of behavioral health integration: evidence update 2010–2015. Milbank Memorial Fund, 2016. Available at: http://www.milbank.org/uploads/documents/Evolving%20Models%20of%20BHI.pdf. Accessed September 10, 2016.

Gilbody S, Bower P, Fletcher J, et al: Collaborative care for depression: a cumulative meta-analysis and review of longer-term outcomes. Arch Intern Med 166(21):2314–2321, 2006 17130383

Guo T, Xiang Y, Xiao L: Measurement-based care versus standard care for major depression: a randomized controlled trial with blind raters. Am J Psychiatry 172 (10):1004–1013, 2015 26315978

Hoeft T, Unützer J: Learning from global mental health research on task shifting to inform the care of older adults in rural and low resource settings. Abstracts from 2015 AAGP Meeting. Am J Geriatr Psychiatry 23(3 suppl):S96, 2015

Katon W, Von Korff M, Lin E, et al: Collaborative management to achieve treatment guidelines. Impact on depression in primary care. JAMA 273(13):1026–1031, 1995 7897786

Katon WJ, Lin EH, Von Korff M, et al: Collaborative care for patients with depression and chronic illnesses. N Engl J Med 363(27):2611–2620, 2010 21190455

Kroenke K, Spitzer RL, Williams JB: The PHQ-9: validity of a brief depression severity measure. J Gen Intern Med 16(9):606–613, 2001 11556941

Kroenke K, Spitzer RL, Williams JB: The Patient Health Questionnaire-2: validity of a two-item depression screener. Med Care 41(11):1284–1292, 2003 14583691

Mauksch LB, Fogarty CT: In search of a perennial philosophy for behavioral health integration in primary care. Fam Syst Health 34(2):79–82, 2016 27270247

Melek S, Norris DT, Paulus J: Economic impact of integrated medical-behavioral healthcare: implications for psychiatry. (Milliman American Psychiatric Association Report) April 2014. Available at: http://psychiatry.org/psychiatrists/practice/professional-interests/integrated-care. Accessed September 10, 2016.

Morris J, Lora A, McBain R, Saxena S: Global mental health resources and services: a WHO survey of 184 countries. Public Health Rev 34:1–18, 2013

Pietruszewski P: A new direction in depression treatment in Minnesota: DIAMOND program, Institute for Clinical Systems Improvement, Bloomington, Minnesota. Psychiatr Serv 61(10):1042–1044, 2010 20889647

Pietruszewski PB, Mundt MP, Hadzic S, et al: Effects of staffing choices on collaborative care for depression at primary care clinics in Minnesota. Psychiatr Serv 66(1):101–103, 2015 25269565

Robinson P, Reiter J: Preface, in Behavioral Consultation in Primary Care: A Guide to Integrating Services. New York, Springer, 2016, p vii

Rossom R, Solberg L, Magnan S, et al: Impact of a national collaborative care initiative for patients with depression and diabetes or cardiovascular disease. Gen Hosp Psychiatry Aug 18, 2016 [Epub ahead of print]

Thomas KC, Ellis AR, Konrad TR, et al: County-level estimates of mental health professional shortage in the United States. Psychiatr Serv 60(10):1323–1328, 2009 19797371

Thota AB, Sipe TA, Byard GJ, et al; Community Preventive Services Task Force: Collaborative care to improve the management of depressive disorders: a community guide systematic review and meta-analysis. Am J Prev Med 42(5):525–538, 2012 22516495

Unützer J: All hands on deck. Psychiatric News, March 3, 2016. Available at: http://psychnews.psychiatryonline.org/doi/full/10.1176%2Fappi.pn.2016.3a28. Accessed September 10, 2016.

Unützer J, Katon W, Callahan CM, et al; IMPACT Investigators. Improving Mood—Promoting Access to Collaborative Treatment: collaborative care management of late-life depression in the primary care setting: a randomized controlled trial. JAMA 288(22):2836–2845, 2002 12472325

Unützer J, Katon WJ, Fan MY, et al: Long-term cost effects of collaborative care for late-life depression. Am J Manag Care 14(2):95–100, 2008 18269305

Unützer J, Chan YF, Hafer E, et al: Quality improvement with pay-for-performance incentives in integrated behavioral health care. Am J Public Health 102(6):e41–e45, 2012 22515849

Von Korff M, Tiemens B: Individualized stepped care of chronic illness. West J Med 172(2):133–137, 2000 10693379

Wagner EH, Austin BT, Von Korff M: Organizing care for patients with chronic illness. Milbank Q 74(4):511–544, 1996 8941260

Whitebird RR, Solberg LI, Jaeckels NA, et al: Effective implementation of collaborative care for depression: what is needed? Am J Manag Care 20(9):699–707, 2014 25365745

Organizational Leadership and Culture Change

Gina B. Lasky, Ph.D., M.A.P.L.

Health care leaders are facing unprecedented change in the way that care is delivered, the goals of the delivery system, and the role of leaders in leading these changes. Leading in the current state of change requires a rich understanding of systems, an engagement of systems leadership, and a foundational appreciation for culture and for leveraging trust to create change. The implementation of the Collaborative Care Model (CoCM) embodies many of the broader shifts in health and health care delivery. Seismic changes in health care include a shift from payment based on volume to payment based on health outcomes, a shift in the locus of control of health from the physician to the individual seeking care, a shift from health occurring in the medical setting to health occurring in the community, a shift from individual health to population health, and a shift from individual health care providers to health care teams. Identifying a leadership model that inspires and facilitates innovation and successful implementation of new models, such as the CoCM, is essential.

Successful development of an integrated approach to health care requires that leadership possess a profound understanding of the culture and organizational evolution involved in the shifts noted above. Every level of the organization will be affected and required to "change practice." Unlike other traditional clinical program additions, collaborative care alters historical and professional identities and well-established and purposeful program boundaries: "a substantial lesson for those working to integrate care is the complexity of it and the time needed to deal with the professional cultural differences encountered when primary care and behavioral health providers begin working together" (Hayes Boober and Ybarra 2015, p. 1). Effective leaders embrace the view that an integrated approach is about facilitating the change in practice (behavior) and is fundamentally grounded in altering beliefs, values, and ultimately identity.

Because of the immense pressure and day-to-day operational challenges that require leadership attention, the time and attention needed for culture change are all too frequently viewed as of secondary importance, "soft" or superficial, time-consuming, distracting from productivity, and/or "touchy-feely." As a result, leaders tend to ignore the broader underlying changes in culture and organization and focus instead on traditional management techniques to execute program implementation. Although these more traditional management techniques are vital to an effective implementation process, they are not sufficient. Leadership interested in a genuine embrace of integration must focus on shifting the foundational levers of change: culture, values, identity, and inspiration.

This chapter begins by outlining the common myths many organizations embrace in the implementation of collaborative care when they do not fully understand or consider the deep and significant impact of change within the collaborative framework. The second section, "Importance of Strong Leadership and Commitment to the Model," provides a model for leadership that is well suited for integrated care and the core elements of transformation needed by health care organizations in meeting the Triple Aim (Berwick et al. 2008). The chapter ends with practical recommendations for leaders on how to avoid the most common mistakes and how to advance models of integration to meet evidence-based components and meaningful outcomes. Case examples and experience from leaders who have successfully built models are also shared.

COMMON ORGANIZATIONAL MYTHS IN IMPLEMENTATION OF COLLABORATIVE CARE

Across the country organizations are embracing integrated care as a method for improving health outcomes, providing a better experience of care, and reducing costs. There is increasing agreement on the problems caused by separate systems of care—particularly medical and behavioral health care. As more organizations implement integrated approaches, consistent themes are arising regarding the challenges and shared myths about the implementation of collaborative care. There are practical reasons for many of these challenges, and the similarities among them highlight the importance of understanding the reasons for why they happen, the techniques for avoiding them, and the impact they have on the long-term success of the model. These are practices that may have worked well up until this point in time; however, the paradigm shift in clinical care requires an equal paradigm shift in leadership and the implementation of best practice.

When leaders decide to engage in health care integration, they make a considerable investment financially and in operational commitment and time. Guaranteeing those resources are used to maximum benefit is a key concern for any leader. For these reasons, a review of the typical challenges faced by those engaged in health care integration can be informative to leaders who are planning for implementation. And during periods of implementation, a review can be even more essential to ensure capitalization of the resources invested.

CoCM Is a Mechanical Change

Organizations often overlook the culture change required to create a fully collaborative care team with a new model of care. This is not simply implementation of another clinical program, but rather a change in the core philosophy of care and a reworking of provider and patient roles and functions within a team approach. The merging of two distinct and siloed cultures— behavioral health and primary care—is complex and a necessary component for building a successful model. In interviews with organizations with successful implementation, leaders often describe one to two previous failed attempts that occurred as a result of ignoring the underlying culture change. In successful implementation, these leaders paid more attention to building the foundation for change and focusing on culture and team development (Lardieri et al. 2014; see also Chapter 3, "Team Development and Culture"). This is not unique to health care or integration but is a consistent finding in literature on ineffective change management. As Kotter describes it, "Smart people miss the mark here when they are insensitive to cultural issues. Economically oriented finance people and analytically oriented engineers can find the topic of social norms and values too soft for their tastes. So they ignore culture—at their peril" (Kotter 2012, p. 38). It may also be that financial change and impact are easier to quantify and thus easier to focus on, whereas quantifying culture change can be far more challenging and, subsequently, easier to ignore.

If We Hire Them, They Will Team

Formal team development is far too often underappreciated. Many leaders believe this "soft" process time is a waste, as well as costly and unproductive. There is a myth that if interdisciplinary providers come together, they will naturally team and function well as collaborative partners, merging roles, training, responsibility, and ultimately culture. The shift in functional power from traditional models of care to integration is huge, and simply co-locating behavioral health providers and primary care providers does not, in and of itself, guarantee integration. It leads instead to "parallel play," in which providers share a space but are not working closely together (Miller et al. 2014). Most providers are not trained in team-based care and thus do not have the attitude or skills to naturally team. Organizational leaders need to believe in and invest in team development, a primary function in culture change (see Chapter 3), if they want effective models.

We Need a Paradigm Shift, But Don't Change Anything

For many organizations, the inclusion of collaborative care stems from the analysis that the current model of care is ineffective, costly, and/or inefficient. The analysis may begin with a realization that behavioral health conditions are contributing to high utilization of expensive services, high disparities including early mortality, reduction in progress on chronic disease management, or challenges with access to traditional behavioral health. Leaders rapidly understand the logic and rational for an integrated approach, and they value the model in part because it is a paradigm shift in the traditional delivery system. However, the mistake that is often made is not accepting the paradigm shift all the way through the process and trying to create a new model while maintaining current staffing ratios and resources. All too common is the desire to "rearrange the deck chairs" rather than to redesign the ship. Leaders are pressured by budgetary constraints and too often try to "pull a rabbit out of a hat," hoping that genuine innovation will occur without having to hire new positions; spend provider time on training, team development, and provider practice changes; and adding resources such as screening tools or operational supports. This generally results in "integration lite" or models that fail to meet evidence-based components and thus miss the targeted outcomes that were the justification and purpose for the change.

Management Is Sufficient

As with many organizational change initiatives, the goal is to successfully manage the implementation process. Although management is an essential element for developing an integrated program, it is not sufficient. In any significant change effort this is true, as Gill points out, "Change efforts that are purely 'managerial' in nature, especially those that are mismanaged, result in a lack of dedicated effort, conflict between functional areas and resistance to change" (Gill 2003, p. 308). Because the nature of the transformation is more significant, the models that have succeeded engage strong leadership in conjunction with effective management techniques. Table 2–1 describes how the lack of clear leadership can influence outcomes.

Clinical Integration Is Enough

CoCM is often misunderstood to be a clinical model that can be implemented similarly to other clinical protocols. Leaders often miss the importance of change for other parts of the system, for example, operational integration such as billing departments who understand physical and behavioral health billing or integrated credentialing. The data needs for the evidence-based model are also important, and thus the integration process occurs within many aspects of the organization and is not simply a clinical activity. In the same way, the leadership approach or "practice" may need to evolve to lead a transformed delivery system.

Like Kryptonite—Pulled to Silo

The strong traditional boundaries between physical health care and behavioral health care are not easily overcome. As organizations shift toward an integrated approach, leaders need to be on their guard for any tendency to drift back toward siloed traditional care. The pull to silo is an ongoing challenge and requires monitoring and action. Without constant vigilance, organizations quickly find themselves with a model that has improved care coordination but remains a traditionally siloed approach to care.

The Jump to False Negative

A common misstep for organizations is choosing metrics that will set the model up for failure. CoCM has a strong evidence base with information on how quickly specific metrics can be met. However, organizations often choose metrics that measure success without consideration of this literature base. As a result, they often choose the wrong metrics or they choose metrics that take time to achieve. When these metrics are not met or not met fast enough, organizations blame the model as a failed approach. For example, the organization presumes that a return on investment will be measured within the first 6 months, or the organization dramatically underresources the behavioral health provider role while expecting the same roles, functions, and achievement of the same outcomes as indicated in the CoCM evidence base.

TABLE 2–1. Consequences of unclear leadership

Reduced participation (among providers)

Lack of clarity about objectives

Low commitment to the quality of care

Limited support for innovation

Increased stress for providers

Source. Summarized from the report of The Effectiveness of Health Care Teams in the National Health Service, a 3-year study investigating how multidisciplinary teams worked together and how team-based care contributes to quality, efficiency, and innovation in health care in the National Health Service (Borrill et al. 1999).

Rushing Through the Starting Gate to Miss the Finish Line

White-water rafters have a saying about safely negotiating a rapid: "It's all in the setup." It is the planning, strategy, and proper placement of the boat in a big rapid that results in success. This is a good metaphor for organizational implementation of integrated care because it requires investment both financially and in time and energy, and the way in which the model is set up has a lasting impact on its longevity and success. Here is the most common mistake for organizations: they decide they want integration, and they rush to get the model up and running with unrealistic time frames that do not allow for proper team development, infrastructure preparation, and training. As a result, these models often miss the promised outcomes, provider satisfaction, and cost savings.

IMPORTANCE OF STRONG LEADERSHIP AND COMMITMENT TO THE MODEL

There are good reasons for the challenges outlined in the previous section of this chapter, "Common Organizational Myths in Implementation of Collaborative Care": genuine integration of behavioral health and primary care is complex and ultimately results in a significant change in organizational culture. Collaborative care demands that organizations overcome historical and entrenched provider silos with separate educational systems and philosophies, often separate funding streams, policy and regulatory differences, and divergent professional cultures. Consequently, leaders are forced to not only lead a health care organization meeting "old-world" rules, regulations, and goals, but to change leadership practice in order to inspire a fundamentally "new world." As a result, leaders are tasked with inspiring their staffs and others with the big picture vision for a new and innovative model while also attending to the nuance of implementation and culture change, including disruption of long-lived hierarchy and power dynamics. In a time when the education system, the practice system, the policy and tort system, and the payment system are all demanding different things and different types of changes, leaders must navigate opposing demands and make clear decisions with genuine commitment.

Research on key components of implementation of integration highlights the importance of leadership in solidifying the interdisciplinary team (Lardieri et al. 2014) and ensuring ultimate model success (Whitebird et al. 2014). Strong organizational leadership provides the foundation for the model, and in the CoCM, research is one of the key components to shifting provider practice and hence changing the clinical model and ultimately health outcomes (Whitebird et al. 2014). Specific leadership components identified in the literature include a commitment to the philosophy of integrated care (John Snow, Inc., and Maine Health Access Foundation 2014; Lardieri et al. 2014); a vision for the model, including specific goals; clarity about the importance of team development (Lardieri et al. 2014); and an ability to articulate and plan for the financial sustainability of the model (Whitebird et al. 2014). As the evaluation of integrated care models matures, consistent evidence indicates that the commitment of leadership is vital to successful implementation. In a recent cross-site evaluation in Maine, the results indicated the following:

> Strong commitment at the leadership level is a key factor for both adoption and implementation of integrated services. If leadership changed, or leadership went on to other priorities, it compromised adoption and implementation of integrated approaches. (John Snow, Inc., and Maine Health Access Foundation 2014, p. 37)

In addition, one of the most important and consistent findings is that these models necessitate a strong interdisciplinary provider team. Individual providers need to act collaboratively and in essence shift from individual values to group or shared values. Provider culture change demands leaders who can create the collective value base. Providers respond to leaders who clearly understand the "dynamic complexity and diversity of specific situations, and the particular needs, desires, intellectual and emotional habits of the persons participating in them" (Bowden 1997, p. 3). Much of the provider change on a collaborative care team is about precisely this—complex behavior change—or breaking of habits, creating new habits, and feeling compelled to act differently.

Strong leaders of successful integrated models appreciate the significance of culture and strongly held values that contribute to providers' deeply ingrained (i.e., trained and practiced) habits. They know that 70% of change initiatives fail (Beer and Nohria 2000), not as a result of poor management but instead because of a lack of effective leadership (Gill 2003). Successful change leadership "requires vision, strategy, the development of a culture of sustainable shared values that support the vision and strategy for change, and empowering, motivating, and inspiring those who are involved or affected" (Gill 2003, p. 307).

Collective values across an organization and team of providers are required for integrated models to be successful and sustainable. Yet the creation of collective values is not simple nor a byproduct of interdisciplinary provider mix. The reality is that interdisciplinary teams are made of individuals who want to maintain their individual values, training, and perspectives. Each provider on the team holds values based on personal beliefs, discipline-specific values, and previous experience as a health care provider. At times any one of these values can be in conflict with the values of another team member and impact the integrated approach to care: "When personal interests outweigh the pursuit of collective values, of what is good for the community at large, value-based practice is derailed" (Prilleltensky 2000, p. 142). To function as a team, there must be a new shared vision that is grounded in shared values that all providers feel inspired and compelled to work toward. Effective collaborative care teams need leaders who understand how to bring "unity from diversity" (M.R. Fairholm, personal communication, May 2015).

Values-Based Leadership

In the existing literature, a few leadership approaches have been described as valuable to building integrated care programs, including transformational leadership, shared or collaborative leadership, boundary spanning leadership, and systems leadership. These models point toward important themes such as a collaborative leadership style, sharing decision-making authority, the ability to span traditional boundaries, and the capacity to see the value of a broader system or collective goal outside a single organization. However, what is missing is a leadership framework that can guide implementation, supporting the big picture vision while also offering specific leadership skills and tasks. Values-based leadership provides this broader framework and is a good fit for changing culture and creating a collective value set.

Values-based leadership is a relational form of leadership that focuses on influencing behavior through values. Leaders "influence others individually and collectively to do or be or think in certain ways" (Fairholm 2013, p. 20). This leadership model emphasizes that "leadership deals with people, individual growth and development, and fostering loyalty and commitment to values, even values held by a group" (Fairholm 2013, p. 21). The consistent evidence that successful CoCM teams had powerful "champions of integration," including primary care provider "champions" and engaged psychiatrists (Whitebird et al. 2014), supports a values-based leader approach. These champions were individuals on clinical teams who innately understood the radical change they were encouraging around them and led the way by demonstrating a commitment to specific values and by successfully influencing others to follow. In many case studies these champions did not have the positional authority to "force" the change; instead, to influence change they engaged in personal relationships with their fellow teammates and thereby revealed the shared values among them.

Finding the points of intersection between behavioral health and primary care cultures and core values is where the sense of a collective whole begins. A leadership model grounded in relationships and the shaping of collective values is precisely what will make integrated models effective.

Create Vision

For values-based leaders, creating a vision is a way to operationalize core values for followers (Fairholm 2013). In an ever-changing health care landscape, a leader's vision must define what makes the team successful and provide the alignment for the many disparate demands of health care policy, financing, and delivery. Leaders need to set the tone and present a vision to ground an organization. Incorporating integrated care into that vision is choosing a model based on values—for example, the value that emotional well-being is important to overall health.

Additionally, an early and central driver of the vision for integrated care was the finding that individuals with serious mental illness were dying 25 years prematurely (Parks et al. 2006). Our collective value of respect for life inspired a vision and compelled action. The status quo was no longer acceptable or congruent with our health care provider core values (equality, respect for humanity, and doing no harm). This kind of value shift allows for culture change and momentum in adopting paradigm shifts in care.

The *value* is what drives behavior and the *vision* is the picture or story that provides the path for change. The significance of a clear and articulated vision has been a consistent theme among studies on integrated care models. Effective leaders provide the team with a clear vision of the model, the interdisciplinary team, and the outcomes of the model (Lardieri et al. 2014). This finding is not a new or surprising understanding about leadership and is based on decades of research on leadership and change management. Creating and inspiring a shared vision is one of the most consistent findings in almost all research on effective leaders; said concisely, "leaders inspire a shared vision" (Kouzes and Posner 2007, p. 17). Leaders are leaders in part because they are individuals who see the future—they have a vision and passion for creating change to obtain the aspiration—they are individuals for whom "their clear image of the future pulls them forward" (Kouzes and Posner 2007, p. 17). Those who achieve their goals are also talented at communicating the idea clearly enough for others to feel inspired and to commit to working toward that vision (Fairholm 2013).

Leaders who compel teams of health care providers to take on challenging behavior change have successfully identified the values underlying the new models. These leaders lead their teams to agreement on those collective values and ultimately to a shared vision for the future: "Vision plays a key role in producing useful change by helping to direct, align and inspire actions on the part of large numbers of people" (Kotter 2012, p. 24). At the same time, these leaders demonstrate humility (shared leadership or even servant leadership) and engage those providers in shaping the specific workflow and in devising solutions that will support the new model and allow innovation on the ground.

"Everyone needs to start from a place of humility and willingness to learn and make a lot of mistakes and know that the way you do the job needs to be different. The whole structure of the organization may change and the way you provide leadership may change."—*Margie Kaems, L.C.S.W., Program Manager, Chambers Hope, Health, & Wellness Clinic, Aurora Mental Health Center, personal communication, January 2015*

When the goals are unclear or an organization is not clear about the problems they are addressing with collaborative care, conflict and disjointed efforts prevent a shift toward integrated care. The term *integrated care* can easily mean different things to different people and therefore needs clear definition for the team. When the vision and model are not clear, it can appear as if the team is working in concert, but in reality each person is reading from a different sheet of music. The CoCM at its core comprises the interwoven actions of all team members, with each member working together in orchestrated concert as a group rather than in disconnected parallel. A clear vision serves as the mechanism (or sheet music) to holistically bring together all team members and their functions.

"Integrated care is a place where you can realize that everyone is on a completely different train in their own minds. It has been shocking."—*M. Kaems, personal communication, January 2015*

Successful leaders will also identify the values of those around them and create a broader vision that aligns with individual values while inspiring a picture of a more rich and meaningful collective value. For example, the identification of a shared value among providers can be leveraged to create a new shared value to inform the model (e.g., measurement of progress)—pushing the providers to the next level and measuring the collective impact of each provider's contribution. Leaders do not ignore individual existing values but build on them and align them in ways that create unity (e.g., both primary care providers and behavioral health providers want to feel that their individual contribution to patient improvement is recognized and important). Rather than simply talking about the vision as an end state, leaders speak directly to individuals' values and beliefs and inspire a different form of commitment and action. Just as the value of the individual patient's perspective is paramount to the team's approach to care, so is the valuing of each individual provider's values and perspective by the leader. As organizations move toward a collaborative care approach, leaders need to continuously find ways to ensure the "actualization of values" is maintained in the implementation of the models (Prilleltensky 2000, p. 141), as this will allow these core values to drive behavior and, essentially, a change in the delivery system. Table 2–2 proposes a connection between value statements and Core Principles of Effective Integrated Care (see Chapter 1, "Elements of Effective Design and Implementation").

Engage Relational Power

Another important reason for values-based leadership in integrated models is that values-based leaders engage power differently—by using relational influence and working with individuals rather than exerting power over others (Fairholm 2013). Kouzes and Posner posit that research on human motivation suggests that extraordinary results occur when individuals are intrinsically motivated—engaged in doing what they want to or doing what pleases them, rather than being forced to act or acting to please others (extrinsic motivation) (Kouzes and Posner 2007, p. 115). Values-based leaders understand that intrinsic motivation is fundamentally connected to values and that influence (power) comes from relationship and shared values:

TABLE 2–2. Value statements underlying the Core Principles of Effective
Collaborative Care[a]

Applying values-based leadership to collaborative care and thinking about
the values underlying some of its core principles, the following represent
potential value-based statements:

- The person receiving care is the most influential and powerful team
  member (person centered).

- We all have a valuable and crucial role to play and share mutual respect
  for one another (team-based care).

- We are better together than we are individually as providers (team-
  based care).

- We have a responsibility to improve people's lives (accountability and
  measurement-based care).

- Do no harm (evidence-based care).

---

[a]For further detail, see Chapter 1, "Elements of Effective Design and Implementation," and https://aims.uw.edu/collaborative-care/principles-collaborative-care.

> What seems to matter more is the kind of relationship or interaction that
> emerges as power is used, and upon that foundation that power is based.... It is
> the relationship that encourages links between people, programs, policies,
> and priorities. (Fairholm 2013, p. 14)

Values-based leaders may have positional authority to "force change";
however, they understand that real change—the kind that is needed to shift
culture and support seminal moments in innovation—requires partnership,
working with individuals, and engaging relational power to inspire, moti-
vate, and compel others.

"The leader treats staff like competent adults who can make decisions and as professionals who have values and can provide
good services rather than acting as a micromanaging person who
tries to make people behave."—*M. Kaems, personal communication, January 2015*

In this way, the leader is demonstrating trust and knowledge of the team
members and what matters most: the value of each team member and the

team's shared values. Strong values-based leaders fundamentally believe in the importance of choice, and they want to influence others to choose to join the movement (Fairholm 2013, p. 14).

ENGAGING VALUES-BASED LEADERSHIP FOR COLLABORATIVE CARE

The following section provides examples of specific leadership activities that can be used to support the development of integrated programs and to bring about the necessary culture change for success. The recommendations are compiled from research on effective change management, evaluations and examples of successful implementation of integrated care models, and leaders who have developed effective programs. The examples and recommendations are presented in three categories: *values, vision,* and *model design and setup*. The expectation is not that all leaders would engage all of these recommendations or that these are a guide for implementation; however, they offer tangible and real-life examples for how to engage values-based leadership for this model of care.

Values

1   Identify the core values underlying the vision for the model and identify ways that as a leader you can demonstrate those core values. For example, be a role model for a nonhierarchical approach to problem solving and be a constant voice for keeping the focus on the population and person at the center of care.

   a. Another consideration is the increasing attention to the joy and satisfaction for providers in their day-to-day work. Bodenheimer and Sinsky (2014) go as far as to argue that care of the provider is the fourth goal of a quadruple aim. For some providers, this may be a central value proposition for changing behavior.

   b. A leader described how identifying core values for the team members allowed them to embrace that value for the population being served. "The space that you provide to listen to our feedback on literally anything we need to bring up about the clinic and also showing that you really want to hear exactly what we are thinking, enables us to provide that same space for the patients we work with" (Margie Kaems, L.C.S.W., Program Manager, Chambers Hope, Health, & Wellness Clinic, Aurora Mental Health Center, personal communication, January 2015).

2. Identify core principles that support the values underlying integrated care and how to build implementation using these principles.

    a. Leaders need to articulate how the CoCM core principles match with the larger value set of the organization and ensure that the model is grounded within a conducive environment (Grantham et al. 2011).

    b. Ensure that the board or governance structure of the organization understands and agrees with the CoCM as a way to act out core values of the organization and is not simply approving the addition of a new clinical program.

3. "Leaders need to invest in adding value and not simply describing values" (Carolyn Shepherd, M.D., Principal, Leibig-Shepherd LLC, personal communication, October 2015). For example, leaders can focus on using their authority to remove barriers that teams encounter. The notion that leaders need to confront obstacles and conflict openly is another tenet of broader change management research—without leadership attention to the barriers, the process of change can be undermined and leave the team feeling disempowered (Kotter 2012).

4. Build leadership infrastructure. An important component of executive leadership leading through values is to support other layers of leadership or management to think through the nuts-and-bolts steps put forward by the value proposition.

    a. "Leaders are there to support the innovation and sustain the change—addressing those harder and way less 'sexy' elements of the work to be sure the organization moves forward" (C. Shepherd, personal communication, October 2015).

    b. Demonstrate the value commitment and willingness to change "leadership practice" to create a new culture. Lead the process of change first and engage management techniques second. Focus on shifting culture within the organization and model so that even executive leadership will be part of the change.

Vision

1. Hold an unwavering commitment to long-term vision of an improved approach to care and demonstrate a genuine understanding of the model and what's required to meet the goals and desired outcomes.

    a. "Administrative and clinical leadership commitment is essential to integrated care implementation success. This includes communication to all staff that integrated care is a priority and allocating sufficient resources for implementation, including staff time. Involving providers in planning will create more buy-in" (Hayes Boober and Ybarra 2015, p. 1).

b. Invest in communication about the model, the vision, and the implementation. This effort may feel like overcommunication; however, "without credible communication, and a lot of it, employees' hearts and minds are never captured" (Kotter 2012, p. 27).

c. A commitment to collaborative care will at times require understanding how the vision is not always aligned with the moving parts of the health care system and a willingness to stay the course with implementation despite perceived risks.

d. While commitment to the vision is imperative, be humble and support innovation and the creation of solutions among care team members. This may require leadership to be open to adjustments for meeting predetermined short-term milestones. Individuals on the front line are best suited to adapt implementation steps and processes.

"Build trust, be transparent, allow constructive disagreement—it is important everyone have a voice and be able to say 'I don't think that will work and here's why.' Team members should be encouraged to share those thoughts and then find solutions."
—*Carolyn Shepherd, M.D., Principal, Leibig-Shepherd LLC, personal communication, October 2015*

---

2. Partner with providers on the front line and staff throughout the organization to find solutions together and to leverage expertise at both the clinical and operational levels in order to develop a strong model.

"Leaders in transformation like collaborative care can get hung up on the idea that they are the innovative person. When there is effective transformation, the leader's role is to create vision but innovation has to come from the people who do the work."
—*C. Shepherd, personal communication, October 2015*

---

3. Engage champions who understand the vision for integrated care and who can also develop relationships with team members to identify and shift provider values from individual to collective team values.

4. Leverage champions to assist with detailed implementation components such as changes to the electronic health record, development of defined

and measurable outcomes (clinical, financial, and patient satisfaction), development of team processes to review data and engage in process improvement, and other elements (Emswiler and Nichols 2009).

5. Define the target population for the CoCM as an essential component for making the vision a reality. Idenfitying a specific population of focus can refine the scope of collaborative care and assist providers in practice change. Agreement on the population of patients that will be served best and designing a specific model for that population clarifies each provider's role and provides a shared problem and a shared goal for the team members, which reduces anxiety and isolation among providers. An example would be deciding to focus on a population of patients with diabetes and depression.

6. Plan for and expect the unexpected. Integrated care is about accepting constant change and constant unpredictability (M. Kaems, personal communication, January 2015). Leaders need to model "holding" a strong and clear vision with flexibility in how that vision becomes a reality, knowing that it may not all go exactly to plan.

7. Plan for and set aside time to talk with the team implementing the model about progress and how the implementation is matching the vision of care. Is the process of implementation tracking with the vision? This commitment to tracking the process and how it evolves is paramount to reaching the identified vision.

Box 2–1 summarizes values-based leadership roles in implementing change.

Box 2–1.   Enabling Successful Complex Change

Higgs and Rowland (2005) describe evidence for a leadership movement shifting from leader-centered and directive approaches to leadership that is facilitative, engaging, and thus enabling. The following are five elements of successful change presented by Higgs and Rowland (2005, p. 127):

1. Creating the case for change: Effectively engaging others in recognizing the business need for change.
2. Creating structural change: Ensuring that the change is based on depth of understanding of the issues and supported with a consistent set of tools and processes.
3. Engaging others in the whole change process and building commitment.

4. Implementing and sustaining changes: Developing effective plans and ensuring good monitoring and review practices are developed.
5. Facilitating and developing capability: Ensuring that people are challenged to find their own answers and that they are supported in doing this.

Promoting the Model Design and Setup

"Good leaders use values-based leadership. They focus on building teams, and the team comes on the path with you because you have demonstrated values-based leadership that assures that they can come with you—trust you. When leaders are absent, organizations struggle, and then midmanagers and frontline staff are blamed for failures when the problem lies in the leadership culture. Being physically present is vital—in person and even in e-mail. You are listening, learning, and hearing what people are saying. You don't have to have the solution but need to demonstrate that discussion is important and help to keep the focus on what is improving care for the patients."—*C. Shepherd, personal communication, October 2015*

Because the lack of an appropriate setup process has been a consistent barrier for effective implementation, as well as the root cause for many later challenges to the model, the model design and setup deserve particular focus. These factors remain important in the implementation and maintenance of the model, and they should be the object of an early focus with maintained attention and development.

"Attention is the currency of leadership. In order to demonstrate importance of a concept (i.e., behavioral health for primary care providers), the leader has to pay attention to behavioral health. In some instances, I personally created the behavioral health staff documentation templates in the computer—not to micromanage the process but to demonstrate the importance of the shift to team care and to ensure inclusion of behavioral health within the primary care setting."—*C. Shepherd, personal communication, October 2015*

1. Communicate the importance of the new model in words, through actions, and with resources. Communication through behavior by the leader is often more powerful than simply through words (Kotter 2012). Keep up the communication and focus for the long term.
2. Invest in culture change through an adaptive change approach and implement solid change management techniques including investment in the resources (time) needed to create change (Hayes Boober and Ybarra 2015).
3. Be present in the setup process and build trust with the team.
4. Support changes to nonclinical operations as part of clinical innovation. This may include changes to the electronic medical record, documentation requirements, consent, productivity standards, scheduling, data systems, and job descriptions and responsibilities across the system (e.g., front-desk staff, finance, credentialing, data, evaluation).
5. Make the implicit explicit. Write down workflows and include every detail of an individual's role—help to build the model explicitly for clarity and to build trust among the team members (C. Shepherd, personal communication, October 2015).
6. Integrate productivity demands with a vision that incorporates new behaviors that support innovation in how services are delivered. Productivity remains essential for any business model and is a reality of quality health care organizations; however, a focus on productivity alone is no longer sufficient.

   a. Increasing evidence from evaluation of successful models shows that organizations need to obtain adequate funding for the start-up of the model. "Start-up funds are essential to pay for nonbillable administrative and clinical personnel time for cross-training, merging professional cultures, changing workflows and protocols, adapting new reimbursement coding and documentation, conducting data and quality of care analysis, and navigating licensing and other regulations" (Hayes Boober and Ybarra 2015, p. 1). This may require added grant funding or other sources to support time and resources required for a sound setup (Grantham et al. 2011).
   b. Consider a brief period of "productivity buffer" or reduced expectations at the beginning of implementation to support the team practicing and engaging in a new model of care. The focus in this phase is development of clear and strong processes that meet the goals of the new model. Examples of time-consuming but essential investments in the setup process include team building, cross-training, changes in workflow, data collection and analysis processes, changes in billing, and other day-to-day operations. Buffered time provides opportunity

for identifying the challenges more quickly and making adjustments that support improved integration more rapidly. In summation, time spent up front may save time and resources in the long run.

7. Create a learning organization culture: "Being a 'learning organization' is an important contextual factor that augments the capacity practices need[ed] in adapting behavioral health practice to the primary care setting. It was also noted as a contextual factor for enhancing leadership commitment, a mechanism that led to successful adoption at the practice level" (John Snow, Inc., and Maine Health Access Foundation 2014, p. 28).

   a. It is important for the leader to promote and support the infrastructure required to support the teams. For example, write out the innovations and ensure that institutional knowledge is retained in the process—both for what works and what fails. Leaders need to instill a culture that engages tracking and documented improvement processes by initially leading the project management, tracking, and documentation that describes organizational learning and accountability (C. Shepherd, personal communication, October 2015).

   b. The learning organization approach models the parallel process for leadership and the clinical team in continuous organizational improvement the same way that teams will be changing practice based on clinical data and outcome metrics in order to engage in continuous improvement.

"When teams wanted to try something new, I would require them to review documentation and summarize previous efforts to address this specific challenge before making the change. They had to go back to the Plan-Do-Study-Act (PDSA) cycles and review findings first. It forced the team members to remember what had been tried before and improve on those attempts rather than repeat them. So often when long-term employees are resistant to change it is because they remember a failed attempt that no one else is validating. It is therefore vital to review previous efforts and to use documentation to capture an organization's learning over time. This is critical to reducing resistance and improving the speed of organizational learning."—*C. Shepherd, personal communication, October 2015*

ADDITIONAL LESSONS FROM THE FIELD

1. Reach out to others; don't be insular.

    a. Engage coaching or other forms of assistance for the team.
    b. Talk with other leaders doing similar work.
    c. Pair with other organizations engaged in similar transformation and share lessons learned.

2. Identify metrics that are realistic. Pushing to meet new goals is important, but staging metrics is also important (see the appendix, "Performance and Outcome Measures for Integrated Care").

    a. Set clear outcomes—both process and health outcomes.
    b. Ensure the chosen outcomes are attainable goals and set new ones as those are reached.
    c. Celebrate milestones.
    d. Be patient with progress.

3. Focus on the "soft stuff" such as team development, and give it the same attention as the "hard stuff."

4. The physical space and setup can affect the speed of collaboration and improve communication within the team. Proximity of providers is essential to improving the integration and collaboration of the care, for example, using cubicle areas as office space for all members of the team rather than separate and discrete office space, or using other shared work space arrangements that facilitate communication among disciplines. Also, placing behavioral health providers near the nurses' station allows them to feel the vibe of the clinic.

5. Maintain the focus, energy, and commitment as success is gained, or as Kotter says, "Consolidate gains and produce more change: premature victory celebration stops all momentum. And then powerful forces associated with tradition take over" (Kotter 2012, p. 35).

6. Spend time in the clinic—learn from those in the trenches.

7. Shadow a patient through the clinic to gain the patient perspective and experience of care.

"Being near each other working made it easy to staff cases and consult. People will learn from each other, and proximity helps blending of cultures—this occurs more rapidly. There was some initial resistance, but it doesn't last as long because you are in the room with all these people."—*M. Kaems, personal communication, January 2015*

RESEARCH FINDINGS ON FACTORS OF EFFECTIVE IMPLEMENTATION

In their study on key care model factors leading to effective implementation of integrated care, Whitebird et al. (2014) discovered several crucial elements related to leadership:

1. Leadership support was significantly related to activating patients into the program.
2. Organizations address financial sustainability—a plan for how to build the model and also a vision with actuarial planning for how to afford the transition leads to stronger models.
3. Leaders' ability to not see operating costs as a barrier was correlated with remission in depression scores. The authors of the research believe this is because it means they offered the CoCM to everyone and were more committed to the outcomes. It could also be that the commitment to offering the model universally demonstrated a genuine commitment and belief in the model, which led to team change and ultimately more consistent change in care for patients.

"Our data show that strong organizational leadership was the most important factor in patient activation; it has long been identified with program success. Providing ongoing institutional support and direction helps lay the foundation on which programs can build. Organizational structure and leadership support are the most common facilitators of success for improving the treatment of depression in primary care. Expert team leadership and support from local management also strongly influence the success of programs for improving depression care." (Whitebird et al. 2014, p. 704)

CONCLUSION

Leaders inspire others. People follow leaders because they believe in the direction, solutions, and values that a leader espouses. Integrated care is a powerful new approach to health care, and it is a paradigm shift that requires real change in the way health care is delivered. Practicing in collaboration shifts our values, changes long-lived habits and behaviors, and forces all of us to stretch beyond entrenched systemic boundaries. Values-based leadership provides a framework for leaders who want to lead this kind of culture transition and presents a mirror image of what provider teams are trying to do with patients—help individuals connect their values to healthy behavior change and then support the choices they make in moving toward a healthier life. Integrated teams cannot "force" or "manage" patients into a healthier life; rather it is the model that engages the patient differently to allow for greater impact and ultimately individual change that results in more healthy choices and behaviors.

Furthermore, as the health care system moves toward value-based outcomes and a focus on quality versus volume of care, there has never been a more important time for strong and principled leadership. Focusing on the big picture and "soft" elements of developing a collaborative care approach can help leaders avoid common pitfalls and lead organizations to improved care with higher-quality outcomes, more satisfied and inspired providers, and ultimately reduced costs.

REFERENCES

Beer M, Nohria N: Cracking the code of change. Harv Bus Rev 78(3):133–141, 216, 2000 11183975

Berwick DM, Nolan TW, Whittington J: The triple aim: care, health, and cost. Health Aff (Millwood) 27(3):759–769, 2008 18474969

Bodenheimer T, Sinsky C: From triple to quadruple aim: care of the patient requires care of the provider. Ann Fam Med 12(6):573–576, 2014 25384822

Borrill C, Carletta J, Carter A, et al: The effectiveness of health care teams in the National Health Service. Aston Centre for Health Service Organization Research, Aston Business School, University of Aston, Human Communications Research Centre, Universities of Glasgow and Edinburgh, and Psychological Therapies Research Centre, University of Leeds. Commissioned by the Department of Health. 1999. Available at: http://homepages.inf.ed.ac.uk/jeanc/DOH-final-report.pdf. Accessed September 10, 2016.

Bowden P: Caring: Gender-Sensitive Ethics. London, Routledge & Kegan Paul, 1997, pp 1–20

Emswiler T, Nichols LM: Baylor Health Care System: High-performance integrated health care. Commonwealth Fund, 2009. Available at: http://www.commonwealthfund.org/~/media/files/publications/case-study/2009/march/baylor-health-care-system/1246_emswiler_baylor_case_study_rev.pdf. Accessed September 12, 2016.

Fairholm MR: Putting Your Values to Work: Becoming the Leader Others Want to Follow. Santa Barbara, CA, Praeger, 2013, pp 1–17, 19–49, 51–77, 91–112

Gill R: Change management—or change leadership? Journal of Change Management 3:307–318, 2003

Grantham S, Coakley E, McKinney A, et al: Integrated behavioral/physical health: a realist evaluation approach. Presented at the 4th annual NIH Conference on the Science of Dissemination and Implementation: Policy and Practice, Bethesda, MD, March 21–22, 2011

Hayes Boober B, Ybarra R: Advancing integrated behavioral health care in Texas and Maine: Lessons from the field. Health Affairs Blog. 2015. Available at: http://healthaffairs.org/blog/2015/08/11/advancing-integrated-behavioral-health-care-in-texas-and-maine-lessons-from-the-field/. Accessed September 12, 2016.

Higgs M, Rowland D: All changes great and small: exploring approaches to change and its leadership. Journal of Change Management 5(2):121–151, 2005

John Snow, Inc, Maine Health Access Foundation: Final evaluation report: Maine Health Access Foundation Integration Initiative: cross-site evaluation of clinical implementation grantees. March 2014. Available at: http://www.mehaf.org/content/uploaded/images/tools-materials/jsi%20final%20report%20march%202014.pdf. Accessed September 12, 2016.

Kotter JP: Leading change. Boston, MA, Harvard Business Review Press, 2012, pp 16–40, 118–145

Kouzes JM, Posner BZ: The Leadership Challenge, 4th Edition. San Francisco, CA, John Wiley & Sons 2007, pp 1–27, 45–73, 103–130

Lardieri MR, Lasky GB, Raney L: Essential elements of effective integrated primary care and behavioral health teams. SAMHSA-HRSA Center for Integrated Health Solutions. 2014. Available at: http://www.integration.samhsa.gov/workforce/team-members/Essential_Elements_of_an_Integrated_Team.pdf. Accessed September 12, 2016.

Miller BF, Petterson S, Burke BT, et al: Proximity of providers: Colocating behavioral health and primary care and the prospects for an integrated workforce. Am Psychol 69(4):443–451, 2014 24820692

Parks J, Svendsen D, Singer P, Foti ME(eds): Morbidity and mortality in people with serious mental illness, Alexandria, VA, National Association of State Mental Health Program Directors (NASMHPD) Medical Directors Council, October 2006. Available at: http://www.nasmhpd.org/sites/default/files/Mortality%20and%20Morbidity%20Final%20Report%208.18.08.pdf. Accessed September 12, 2016.

Prilleltensky I: Value-based leadership in organizations: balancing values, interests, and power among citizens, workers, and leaders. Ethics Behav 10(2):139–158, 2000

Whitebird RR, Solberg LI, Jaeckels NA, et al: Effective implementation of collaborative care for depression: what is needed? Am J Manag Care 20(9):699–707, 2014 25365745

CHAPTER 3

Team Development and Culture

Gina B. Lasky, Ph.D., M.A.P.L.

EFFECTIVE COMPONENTS OF COLLABORATIVE CARE TEAMS ARE NOT NEW

A core principle of the Collaborative Care Model (CoCM) is that treatment occurs through patient-centered team-based care (see Chapter 1, "Elements of Effective Design and Implementation"). In fact, the collaboration between team members and patients is at the heart of the model and central to the broader mission of achieving improved team outcomes, improved quality of experience, reduced costs, and ultimately population health.

Team effectiveness has received decades of investigation across numerous disciplines, such as social psychology and psychology, business management, organizational development, and professional sports. National policy (see Chapter 7, "Policy and Regulatory Environment"), practice innovation, and the desire to contain costs are driving a renewed emphasis on health care teams and subsequently a dismantling of hierarchical structures and singular provider practice. Consistent research, such as findings that members of effective teams have higher job satisfaction and are more efficient in achieving shared goals, goes back decades (Levi 2017; Wheelan 2013) and is currently an important element of health care transformation: "The high-performing team is now widely recognized as an essential tool for constructing a more patient-centered, coordinated and effective health care delivery system" (Mitchell et al. 2012, p. 3).

Evidence of this broad shift includes a focus by the Institute of Medicine on the development of effective health care teams and even more broadly the concept of "transdisciplinary professionalism" that emphasizes cross-disciplinary accountability (Cuff 2014; Mitchell et al. 2012). Further interest in this approach is suggested by the investments and shifts from big industry in health care to create teams (e.g., Kaiser Permanente's announcement about opening a medical school to specifically train providers in an integrated system approach with an emphasis on how to practice on care teams) and growing evidence that desired outcomes and cost savings arise with approaches that are team based (Bodenheimer 2003; Katon et al. 2012; Melek et al. 2012; Missouri Department of Mental Health and MO Health Net 2013; Shortell et al. 2004; Reiss-Brennan et al. 2016).

Creating effective integrated teams requires more than simply putting interdisciplinary team members in a single clinical setting. Instead, development of a team entails a shift from individual practice that may be coordinated or in concert with other providers to an authentic team-based approach at each phase of the treatment process. Creating this authentic team requires culture change and establishing effective group norms (Wheelan 2013). Group norms consist of the formal (clearly articulated) and informal rules (unconscious and unspoken but known) of the team. Team norms provide four main functions for teams: 1) giving the team a sense of who they are (core values of the team); 2) setting expectations on the work or activities of the team, which ensures some predictability of behavior; 3) providing boundaries around appropriate behavior, which creates psychological safety (Edmondson 1999) and thus an ability to participate in the team; and 4) setting the identity of the team (Levi 2017).

Although establishing norms sounds intuitive or even organic, the reality of fostering an effective team culture is not. Boon and colleagues (2004) outline a continuum of seven types of health care teams (i.e., parallel, consultative, collaborative, coordinated, multidisciplinary, interdisciplinary, integrative), noting change along the continuum of collaboration in philosophy of care, structure of the team, process components, and outcomes. This chapter outlines the importance of pointed, purposeful, and thoughtful development of the team and the norms that are the foundation for an effective integrated care team. Effective teams share a common set of core components that individuals on teams can articulate and that research has demonstrated improve team functioning.

ORGANIZATIONAL LEADERSHIP COMMITMENT TO TEAM DEVELOPMENT

An *integrated health care team* has been defined as "the care that results from a practice of primary care and behavioral health clinicians, working together with patients and families, using a systematic and cost-effective approach to provide patient-centered care for a defined population" (Peek and National Integration Academy Council 2013, p. 2). Using Boon et al.'s (2004) framework, health care innovation is a change in philosophy of care to whole person care in one setting, a new interdisciplinary team structure, a different workflow and emphasized team processes, and a focus on tracking metrics to improve the team's ability to treat to target.

As discussed in Chapter 2, "Organizational Leadership and Culture Change", creating effective and successful teams with this kind of culture change requires organizational leaders who believe in and understand the need for concerted time, resources, and unique leadership. This organizational context impacts team effectiveness by influencing the initial conditions that do or do not promote functionality (Lemieux-Charles and McGuire 2006). Far too often, however, team development is deemed the "soft stuff" and subsequently receives inadequate organizational attention. The outcome of that decision is a poor team culture and challenges with obtaining expected outcomes.

In actuality, team development is far and away the "hard stuff" or, as a colleague likes to say, "the strong stuff" of integrated care, as it is in any industry. In a recent study on internal team effectiveness outside the field of medicine, the information technology company Google found that above all other factors, a team's "psychological safety" was important to effectiveness (Duhigg 2016). Psychological safety is a component of team culture that allows for taking interpersonal risk because there is an absence of judgement or shame when individuals share ideas; psychological safety has also been found to support learning in organizations (Edmondson 1999). What Google is demonstrating is how team leaders who foster and attend to this team process can directly impact the success of the organization.

For collaborative care, the same early emphasis and focus on team development is required by leaders, including nudging providers to embrace an identity shift and sacrifice some of the trained and long-ingrained patterns of individual practice. Creating a team that embraces psychological safety and a culture of collaboration requires early and ongoing energy and resources. These are not simply mechanical changes, such as the number of people on the team or new processes, but a real embrace of new group norms and ultimately culture. Providers are often comfortable with the status quo, which can inadvertently maintain their investment in traditional models of roles, responsibilities, infrastructure, systems, beliefs, and assumptions. In traditional models, providers share an understanding of the model with all disciplines "speaking their unique languages" and sharing expectations of hierarchy. These are historical health care team norms, and dismantling them and establishing new expectations of behavior are at the root of collaborative care and the effectiveness that arises from a different philosophy. The new team norms expect providers to embrace learning and the sharing of languages, new processes, new goals of treatment, and, most importantly, a new identity. Culture is a powerful force, and therefore any effort to change culture must include exponential resources for change to gain traction.

PAINTING A PICTURE OF INTEGRATED TEAMWORK

Collaborative care teams function differently than other forms of interdisciplinary health care teams. The degree of integration and collaboration means care is delivered through a shared approach, shared activities, and shared space.

Shared Definition of the Problem

Collaborative care teams have shared goals in part because they share a conceptualization of the problem. They believe in the need for whole person care, and they have experienced the challenges associated with siloed medical and behavioral health care. Collaborative care teams may not always immediately agree on all specific elements of the care plan or a patient's presentation, but team members share the perspective that both medical and behavioral health conditions play a role in the plan.

Case Example

A primary care provider (PCP) is working with a young woman who is complaining of poor sleep and is requesting "sleeping pills." The PCP consults with the behavioral health provider (BHP) and learns that the husband of this patient routinely comes home late at night and is abusive to the patient who then has trouble sleeping. Understanding the problem and sharing the root cause made all the difference in this case, as sleeping medication was not an adequate solution.

Shared Activities and Space

Team members may provide an intervention together with a patient or even start an exam together, and they share team space for documentation, discussion, and planning for the day.

Case Example

An individual with serious mental illness (bipolar disorder) came in for her first well-woman visit in over 50 years. The PCP entered the room and immediately exited, saying to the BHP, "I can't see this patient." The BHP inquired why and learned that the patient had disrobed in the exam room, was talking loudly to herself, and scrubbing the sink." The BHP calmly said to the provider, "We can do this together," and they returned together to the room and completed this important exam.

This example highlights that the team members' tasks may have been different (the PCP had a physical exam to perform and the BHP leveraged calming and engaging techniques to assist the patient with behavioral health symptoms) but the goal was shared, the space was shared, and the positive outcome was shared with the patient. This quality care experience necessitated a team approach.

Shared Decision Making

Shared decision making is a hallmark of integrated teams and one of the elements of effective health care teams (Kinman et al. 2015). Team members also share decision making with the patient. Integrated team members work together to make decisions, informing each other of relevant aspects of the individual's health and deciding on a course of action as a group. Underlying this ability is an appreciation for each other's skills and knowledge and a genuine commitment to collaboration over individual practice. At the same time, teams still maintain clear moments of defined accountability appropriate with licensure and scope of practice in decision making. For example, a PCP decides on a course of action that is critical to a medical condition; however, the decision is shared with the team and there is mutual respect and incorporation of other components of care that are informed by other team members' expertise. In a review of health care team effectiveness, the authors summarized their findings this way: "[The] type and diversity of clinical expertise involved in team decision making largely accounts for improvements in patient care and organizational effectiveness" (Lemieux-Charles and McGuire 2006, p. 263).

Case Example

In a pediatric collaborative care clinic, the pediatrician raised concerns about a young girl (around 15 years old) who was morbidly obese and developing significant heart disease. The pediatrician was highly distressed about the girl and her medical condition, and she expressed concern that she was failing to create enough urgency for the patient and the family to make significant behavior changes. The pediatrician expressed life-and-death concern for this patient and suggested that the BHP do a number of tasks, all directed at "forcing" the family to change. The BHP, however, suggested an alternative approach for engaging the patient and the family and provided important background about the parents that the pediatrician was unaware of. Through discussion, the team members created a collaborative approach with the pediatrician, BHP, and nurse, each having a clear role with the patient and her family. The medical decision about the course of action was made by the pediatrician, but the approach and solution to get to the shared goal was made as a team. Part of the BHP's plan also incorporated how to engage the family in deciding how they wanted to approach the treatment, giving some of the shared decision making back to the patient and family.

Shared Responsibility and Outcomes

Directly related to shared decision making is shared responsibility for the care and ultimately the outcomes. Even if one member of the team is more responsible for the interventions, the solution and care plan are agreed to by the team. Conflicts or disagreements about the approach are worked out, and the patient's preferences and input are part of the process. The team, not individual providers, are then responsible for the outcomes.

Teams that are able to share and integrate in these ways have similar core components, all of which were part of their setup or developmental process. These core components focus on team composition, formal and informal team development, system and operational supports, and outcomes.

TEAM COMPOSITION

Collaborative care teams are made up of medical providers (physicians, nurse practitioners, and physician assistants), BHPs (usually licensed clinical social workers or doctoral-level psychologists; see Chapter 4, "Behavioral Health Provider Essentials"), nurses, and medical assistants. Also central to the team is the psychiatric consultant (see Chapter 6, "The Psychiatric Consultant") who is actively engaged but usually not physically present day to day. Other team members can include pharmacists, nutritionists, peer specialists, and/or community health workers or other team members depending on the clinical setting. In addition, these teams have organizational leaders, clinic managers, and other operational and supportive team members from quality improvement, billing, medical records, and information technology.

As teams are developed, consideration of each individual's personality traits is a vital factor. There has been extensive research on team member traits that tend to improve team functioning. The Institute of Medicine describes the personal values most associated with effective health care teams: honesty, discipline, creativity, humility, and curiosity (Mitchell et al. 2012). Other authors have found mutual respect among team members to be a central characteristic for contributing to highly effective health care teams (Mickan and Rodger 2005).

Because member traits impact teaming, carefully selecting and hiring the right people is important. Not all providers thrive in integrated models. There are medical providers and BHPs who prefer traditional models of care and who will resist practice change. As a result, gauging a potential team member's interest in the model is essential, as well as looking for individuals who are good team players, flexible, willing to experiment and learn, enjoy creative problem solving, and are passionate about a new model. Additionally, exploring a person's communication skills and willingness to disengage from traditional medical hierarchies is worthwhile. Exploring personality traits in the interview process is one avenue to evaluate fit (see Chapter 4). See Box 3–1 for troubleshooting challenges once a team has been formed.

Box 3–1. When a Team Member Is Not a Team Player

Some employees work best independently and do not thrive on a team. This presents a dilemma for leadership, especially when skilled professionals are in short supply. The team should be given an opportunity to voice their solutions for this problem, as these situations can make teamwork difficult and ineffective. Questions to consider:

✓ Is the team able to share the workload if the team is short-handed in the event that this person moves off the team?
✓ Is a coach available to provide training for specific behavioral changes to improve teamwork?
✓ Is there another position for the person in the organization that would be a better fit?
✓ Is there someone else in the organization that may not be highly experienced but is highly motivated to join a team and with support could transition into the needed position?

Team Champion

In addition to specific characteristics for providers, there is a distinct role for a team champion or champions. Building a team with a champion is both useful for leadership and productive for the team. Champions can be PCPs or other members of the team (BHPs are often the champions, as discussed in Chapter 4; and psychiatric consultants play a role here as well, as indicated in Chapters 6). Regardless of their specific role, champions are passionate about the model and about team-based care and often hold the team accountable to the core principles. A champion's investment in the transition and the model is instrumental in facilitating culture and practice change, and there is evidence that the presence of a champion on a team improves perceived team effectiveness (which is related to improved outcomes; Shortell et al. 2004). Furthermore, Whitebird et al. (2014) found that a strong physician champion and an engaged psychiatrist were essential for patient activation and reaching remission in the CoCM.

Team Leaders

As discussed in Chapter 2, organizational leaders play a vital role in creating effective integrated teams (Cohen et al. 2015). Organization leaders create a broader culture and environment that promote collaboration; they provide the resources and time needed to foster a sense of team; and they commit organizational resources that support the new clinical approach.

Leadership at the team level is also an important consideration. Although these teams are by definition collaborative, by no means are the teams leaderless. In fact, most teams have clear leaders who may be the physician lead for the clinic or another organizational manager who works directly on the team. In smaller organizations, the team leader may in fact be the organizational leader (e.g., CEO). Some teams have a more formal leadership structure, whereas others engage in shared leadership; however, all teams have the shared value of collaboration. What matters is that the team members embrace a team approach:

> Notions of independent practice were not relevant because no one member of the team was seen as practicing alone, and leadership questions were not sources of conflict; rather, when leadership issues were raised they were portrayed as matters for open discussion that led to mutually agreeable solutions. (Mitchell et al. 2012, p. 12)

Additionally, team leaders who cultivate inclusiveness (both in spirit and in action) can assist teams in overcoming hierarchical status and improve psychological safety, ultimately facilitating team member engagement and quality care (Nembhard and Edmondson 2006).

These more "on the ground leaders" are the primary designers of the team scaffolding (Valentine and Edmondson 2014), including team member roles and team structures. In a review of exemplary integrated behavioral health and primary care teams, Cohen et al. (2015) found that this kind of scaffolding "meant striking a balance between structure (clear roles and responsibilities, protocols) and the flexibility that was needed for integrated care teams to function effectively" (p. 57). Building team scaffolding that promotes communication, shared accountability, a sense of group identity and belonging, and clarity about where team member work overlaps is important (Valentine and Edmondson 2014). Yet integrated care teams also thrive on the flexibility to be creative and to leverage the team's expertise as needed. Effective team leaders provide structure to help the team define clear roles and responsibilities and to manage task sharing, while also ensuring that team members practice at the top of their license to improve efficiency. At the same time, the team leader relies on innovation and solutions from team members, engaging in the same openness to process improvement as the team does with patient and outcome feedback. Team leaders can also be an objective voice for the team by helping the team with their incorporation of information, thereby improving and fostering reflection and examination of team processes. Most importantly though, leaders recognize the incredible value and richness of formal team development and the process of creating and maintaining a collaborative team.

FORMAL AND INFORMAL TEAM DEVELOPMENT

Both formal and informal team development are essential for building effective teams in integrated care.

Formal Team Development

Team development is essentially a focused pursuit of culture change. It is the design phase for the elements and structures that support the shift from individual provider units to a functioning and effective team. As the initial development process, formal team development provides the foundation for shared actions (described in the section "Team Composition" earlier in this chapter) and facilitates the collaboration and integration of team member expertise. When functioning in traditional silos, traditional medical providers and BHPs have the following differences in the culture of treatment approach:

- Goals of care (continuity vs. termination or discharge)
- Treatment of patient data (shared vs. private)
- Panel sizes (small vs. large)
- Scheduling (flexible vs. fixed) and cadence of care (fast paced vs. slower paced)
- Boundaries (flexible vs. firm)
- Disease models (disease management vs. recovery) (see Raney 2015 for more detail)

As a result of these differences, team development is first and foremost focused on creating a new and shared culture.

Shared Values

The importance of shared values to high-functioning teams is well established (Kinman et al. 2015; Mitchell et al. 2012; Wheelan 2013). As integrated care teams are formed, it is important for these teams to explicitly define shared values around the philosophy of care, the commitment to a team approach, and other values that may help the team connect to the broader organizational mission. For example, some teams articulate a shared value and understanding of patient-centered care or quality patient care for a specific population, whereas other teams may focus on equality in care or reduction of health disparities. The value set provides the underlying reason or vision for integration. These fundamental values about the purpose of the care can assist teams in making difficult choices about treatment for individuals and serve to reduce conflict among team members (Lardieri et al. 2014). Explicit values are also significant in shaping group norms and help team members hold each other accountable to norms in a nonthreatening manner.

Shared Goals

After defining values, teams need to choose specific shared goals.

> The foundation of successful and effective team-based health care is the entire team's active adoption of a clearly articulated set of shared goals for both the patient's care and the team's work in providing that care. (Mitchell et al. 2012, p. 6)

For integrated teams, three levels of shared goals are often identified: 1) goals that articulate the team's vision or broad based goals, 2) shared goals for specific health outcomes for the defined population, 3) and process goals that are about how the team will function. Box 3–2 provides an example of these three levels of goals.

Box 3–2.   Example of Shared Goals at Three Levels

1. **Vision or broad goal:** Reduce health disparities for individual with behavioral health conditions.
2. **Specific health outcome goal:** Include a treat-to-target metric, such as 80% of the patient population will have controlled diabetes.
3. **Process goal:** The team will engage in the following activities to reach the health outcomes: universal screening, tracking of behavioral health and physical health metrics within a reg-

istry, reviewing progress as a team, and a commitment to on-going cross-training.

All three levels of goal setting provide a road map for how the team will measure success. In fact, research demonstrates the following:

> The clearer the team's objectives, the higher the level of participation in the team, the greater the emphasis on quality and the higher the support for innovation, the more effective the team was reported to be by its members and external raters. (Mickan and Rodger 2005, p. 212)

Roles and Responsibilities

"Diversity of expertise underpins the idea of effective teams" (Interprofessional Education Collaborative Expert Panel 2011, p. 20). As a core principle, team-based care acknowledges that improved care stems from combining different perspectives, forms of expertise, and knowledge about treating the human condition. The evidence is clear that when separated in traditional care models, no medical discipline can achieve the same degree of quality and population health as when diversity of expertise is combined.

Yet, team-based care does not eliminate important differences in team member functions or scope of practice considerations. Rather, effective teams utilize the team approach to ensure that each individual practices within their scope of practice and at the top of their license or credentials (i.e., reserving the time of licensed staff for potentially billable services). However, by being more knowledgeable about the other team members' skill sets and having shared goals, the team can add functions and elements of care that are generally missed in traditional practice (i.e., enhancing patient activation, incorporating solutions for social needs, and addressing the interaction of behavioral and medical symptoms). Understanding how to combine skill sets in order to maximize resources to meet shared goals is one of the key advantages of team-based care. "Effective coordination and collaboration can occur only when each profession knows and uses the others' expertise and capabilities in a patient-centered way" (Mitchell et al. 2012, p. 20).

As a result, integrated care teams need to spend time early on learning each other's strengths, skills, and knowledge base. For example, often medical providers are unaware of the degree to which licensed clinical social workers have expertise in diagnosis and treatment of behavioral health conditions and are not simply experts in social service resource allocation. Spending time in the formation phase to enhance this knowledge can build efficiency later on in the practice of integrated care. A PCP's understanding of the depth of the

BHP's expertise can reduce the PCP's desire to bypass the BHP and can reduce unnecessary contacts with the psychiatric consultant (see Lardieri et al. 2014 for examples of how to build this awareness between providers).

Once team members are aware of what each member brings to the team, the next step is to formalize the role and functions that each team member will play to ensure that specific components are addressed and there is a clear understanding among team members regarding each function (e.g., screening, scoring, alerts to specific team members, updates to patient). This step may occur in general in designing the approach to care, but it may also have variation with daily staffing changes. The Advancing Integrated Mental Health Solutions (AIMS) Center at the University of Washington offers a useful workflow plan worksheet to break down functions for assignments (see http://aims.uw.edu/resource-library/clinical-workflow-plan).

A team that spends time thinking through model components and functions during team development will be more effective and able to adapt roles as needed. Without clear role assignments, planned model components may be overlooked, delayed, or left undone when specific team members are absent. The most common example occurs when one individual is assigned behavioral health screening, and then when this individual is not available screening comes to a halt. A team approach to owning and designing all functions helps to prevent separation of vital components while maintaining clarity of individual roles.

Similarly, it is important to distinguish between title and function on the team. Teams can become mired in traditional boundaries, dividing up team member functions based on titles or disciplines, which can inappropriately limit flexibility and effectiveness when functions cross disciplines. For example, a common mistake is to say that any education provided to a patient about behavioral health concerns must be completed by the BHP. Often basic education can be delivered by the PCP, the registered nurse, or other team members such as health navigators or peers. Breaking down roles and responsibilities into specific functional tasks is therefore an important process in assisting the team with seeing the variety of ways each individual team member can play a role and with defining when specific knowledge or licensure status will need to be engaged. All of the time spent on overtly defining these components helps to ensure team efficiency, as well as accountability and clarity for team members. See Chapter 4 for an example of how the BHP's role can be divided into specific tasks and shared across team members.

Role of the Patient

Another role to consider is that of the patient. Integrated care teams are patient centered, with the patient's goals defining the treatment approach. Patient-centered teams have been found to be more effective (Shortell et al. 2004). However, being truly patient centered takes effort.

> In high-functioning health care teams, patients are members of the team, not simply objects of the team's attention; they are the reason the team exists and the drivers of all that happens. (Wynia et al. 2012, p. 1327)

Patients can be engaged in many ways as team members in integrated care, with the primary role of the patient being to set goals and identify priority treatment needs as well as to share in decision making about treatment choices. Shared decision making recognizes that both clinical providers and patients may view options differently and that both viewpoints are important to determining the best course of action (Coulter and Collins 2011). Forging a new reality of shared decision making requires that clinicians provide patients with the evidence and risks of treatment and that patients and family provide clinicians information on what's most valued in the patient's life and how decisions may impact those life goals. For both patients and medical providers accustomed to traditional care, making collaborative decisions is a new skill.

Engaging patients and family members in reviewing treatment options and incorporating those choices into providers' own value sets is enhanced by teams with diverse expertise. The mixture of team members' skills in evidence-based care and risk management combined with expertise in motivational interviewing and patient engagement can improve goal setting and discussion around challenging treatment decisions. BHPs may be particularly useful to patients in ensuring that they understand the information and in helping individuals make decisions based on their current readiness for change and their goals. It is important that during team development, members review the role of the patient and that patients are given information about roles and responsibilities as they enter an integrated treatment program.

A secondary role for patients is that of providing valuable feedback to the treatment team on how the integrated approach is working or not working, which offers valuable insight into patient satisfaction. Shortell et al. (2004) found that teams with greater patient satisfaction also have greater perceived team effectiveness (which can result in improved outcomes). Engaging patients in providing feedback on their experience is not only essential to patient centeredness but may in fact improve the likelihood of the team meeting its goals.

Patients in a clinic played a vital role in improving processes by highlighting that it was hard to work with a team when multiple team members called them (often on the same day) regarding outcomes or findings (e.g., depression screening, lab work, diabetes registry). Patients were highlighting both a failed communication among team members but also an existing team approach that ultimately was not patient centered.

Cross-Training

Another core component of formal team development is cross-training. One of the significant advantages to an interdisciplinary team is the ability to improve team members' skills and capacity. Although knowledge transfer occurs often through osmosis and merely being in each other's presence, "rubbing elbows" and exchanging expertise, it is important in formal team development to set the tone for this cross-fertilization. The goal is to improve team member knowledge across domains and enhance everyone's acquisition of new skills. Each team needs to determine the specific topics of cross-training; however, most collaborative care teams address a core set of topics, including signs, symptoms, and treatment targets for common diagnoses (medical and/or behavioral). Medical providers can train other team members on the signs and symptoms of chronic disease and important self-management skills, as well as metrics to determine progress. BHPs can teach team members about behavioral health conditions, including signs and symptoms, as well as effective treatment and communication approaches. Psychiatric consultants provide case-based and didactic training on diagnosis and treatment, including evidence-based psychopharmacology. Other common topics for cross-training include how to take "integrated vitals" (e.g., blood pressure, body mass index), how to use behavioral health screening tools, and how to provide specific evidence-based techniques and interventions, such as motivational interviewing and behavior activation.

It is important for this cross-training to occur during team development; however, training should be ongoing and should become a way for the team to improve sophistication of treatment for specific challenges that the population raises (e.g., methods for reducing stigma around obesity, education on specific trends in substance use, engaging individuals in tobacco cessation, improving patient engagement and active shared decision making; see Box 3–3). Teams with peer specialists or community health workers can take advantage of training opportunities to learn more about population-specific needs, patient-centered language, and other factors specific to the community being served.

Box 3–3. The Importance of Cross-Training

"[We] found out very quickly that we weren't even speaking the same language. Abbreviations are different, etc. For example, 'MI': [behavioral health providers] are talking about motivational interviewing and I'm talking about a heart attack! Very different....Getting on the same page, talking the same language, understanding how we practice, and what we do when we see a patient [are] very different things. [We spend] a lot of time just talking to each other and cross-training. We'd do a presentation of diabetes basics and how we manage them for the health coach, and then I'd get a presentation on dialectical behavioral therapy. Learning from each other and bringing in some outside experts to teach the team as a whole— it was six months together in the group learning these things about each other and learning each other's focus before we ever saw a patient." (Lardieri et al. 2014, p. 16; *the experience as described by a medical provider at Cherry Health in Michigan*)

Workflow and Process Formation

As Boon et al. (2004) outlined, team processes change as health care teams become more integrated. In addition to incorporating new team members (BHP and psychiatric consultant) to primary care, collaborative work requires significant changes in clinical processes, including the workflow. The change in workflow is often the hardest element for teams to comprehend before starting the model, which highlights the importance of spending time clearly defining process changes during team development. Each team will find the specific and unique workflows that facilitate inclusion of BHPs, and challenges can be avoided by giving the team opportunities to think through the best approach together. The following sample workflow and process components should be determined:

- Purpose and format of team huddle
- Development of screening protocols, including cadence of rooming patients
- Definition of warm handoffs (see Chapter 4), including scripted introductions
- Purpose and format of team meetings
- Process for when and how data and metrics will be routinely reviewed

Box 3–4 provides tips for the BHP role in team development.

Box 3–4.   The BHP Role in Team Development

Because the addition of a BHP is one of the new team members in integrated models, BHPs play a unique role in team development. As outlined in Chapter 4, the BHP is truly the heart of the model. BHPs have training in culture change, building effective group norms, and team process. As a result, BHPs impact the development of the team and are the key member to maintain the team's focus on further development. Specifically, the BHP does the following:

✓ Reminds the team to include behavioral health at all phases of care.
✓ Reminds the team of core model components and alerts the team when these are missed.
✓ Facilitates and promotes communication across the team and keeps pressure on the team to incorporate new processes such as new workflows or procedures (e.g., warm handoffs, registry review, screening).
✓ Keeps patient goals at the center of team focus.
✓ Facilitates and monitors progress and data for the team.
✓ Brings data to the team to review and utilize to inform treatment decisions.
✓ Translates culture between patient, medical, and behavioral health, as well as additional members of the team.

Informal Team Development

In addition to formal team development, other factors support the foundation of strong teams. These factors may be considered facets of informal team development because they are less structured at times but still are impactful in forming the culture of a team. The most important task of informal team development is to provide opportunities for the team members to get to know one another as people and to build relationships that are not purely based on work. Teams may have lunch together, have monthly dinners, or even more structured outings such as bowling (see Lardieri et al. 2014 for additional examples). Getting to know each other as people facilitates a team's relationships and their ability to work together. Although these seemingly social gatherings are often underappreciated by leaders, many team members describe these opportunities as essential to team development.

"Building positive relationships between staff members is so critical, because this is often the foundation that helps them to see the common values we hold in the helping profession, and then we can blend the cultures."—*Margie Kaems, L.C.S.W., Program Manager, Chambers Hope, Health, & Wellness Clinic, Aurora Mental Health Center, personal communication, January 2015*

Another factor to consider in informal team development includes space considerations and how to enhance opportunities for "hallway conversations" or "curbside consultations" that allow planned or unplanned team member communications. If team members have separate offices with doors, there is less opportunity to consult with one another or spontaneously share information about patient care. Many integrated care teams have found that a centralized team room, a shared nurses' station for documentation, or even cubicle office space rather than traditional offices improves team communication and relationships. Regardless of the specific space, many of these team members report that the shared space facilitates team communication, patient care planning, cross-provider education, advancement in knowing each other's skills and roles on the team, and just getting to know each other as people. As one team member stated, "You learn to know what your team members like to eat, what makes them laugh, and how to improve a bad day." Many organizations are designing new facilities with this interactive space in the design.

TEAM PROCESS

With a solid foundation of development, the team has strong scaffolding and can use day-to-day processes and structures to institutionalize elements initiated during formal team development. Team process components are the supports that maintain collaboration and long-term effectiveness. Regular attention to these forms of ongoing team development enhances the model of care and ensures that the model remains consistent with the core principles.

Communication

By far the most important process component to focus on for cohesive and effective teams is communication. Effective communication is central to team success and "should be considered an attribute and guiding principle of the team, not solely an individual behavior" (Mitchell et al. 2012, p. 16). Team members need to let each other know they have a readiness for working together, shown in several of the following ways: "being available in place, time and knowledge, as well as being receptive through displaying interest, engaging in active listening, conveying openness, and being willing to discuss [concerns or questions]" (Interprofessional Education Collaborative Expert Panel 2011, p. 22). High-functioning teams foster a culture of open communication that supports any team member in expressing thoughts and engaging in interpersonal risk taking (Edmondson 1999; Wheelan 2013) while avoiding the misuse of status or hierarchy. This approach requires a shared language that is free from excessive professional jargon (which can alienate team members) and exhibits an underlying foundation of mutual respect. This is not synonymous with permitting only harmonious communication; in fact, conflict is an important element of team effectiveness. Rather, constructive conflict among high-functioning team members is brief and managed with effective conflict resolution skills (Wheelan 2013).

In integrated models, there are multiple categories and functions of communication, such as huddles, clinical case review, day-to-day treatment and operational planning, and team process. Each type of communication may be supported by specific tools, such as the following:

• **Clinical case review** generally occurs during registry review or team meetings when more time can be devoted to discussion about treatment approach, although some teams include brief case presentations within their daily huddle.
• **Day-to-day clinical and operational communication** includes brief clinical updates, schedule review, and logistics planning. The day-to-day treatment and operational planning is primarily supported by huddles (see the section "Huddle" later in this chapter) with additional support from electronic medical record messaging, alerts, e-mail, phone calls, and "hallway" conversations. Some members of the team may also use various communication tools more than others; for example, the BHP and psychiatric consultant communicate most often via the phone.
• **Team process communication** is discussion about how the team is working together and occurs throughout the day in brief feedback sessions; however, team process communication is generally more fully addressed in a regular team meeting with routine review of team processes and procedures, data on process and health outcomes, and arising innovations or adjustments to advance care.

Teams often create their own supportive tools for communication, such as a scripted huddle or case presentation, a standing agenda for team meetings that sets an expectation of team process review, and a leveraging of technology in a way that is best suited for the team. A well-known tool for teaching team members shared clinical presentation skills is the Situation, Background, Assessment, and Recommendation (SBAR) technique, which is a standardized way to present patient information quickly. Tools such as SBAR help to frame team member conversations and allow all team members a shared understanding of what to expect as well as what information to include. For example, BHPs are trained in case presentation with a heavy emphasis on patient history, whereas medical providers will deem training in this history as unnecessary. Tools such as SBAR can assist team members on focusing on the most important clinical factors to share. Shaping the team's specific clinical presentation format happens over time as BHPs, PCPs, and psychiatric consultants share with one another what information they need in order to be able to move forward with treatment.

Team leaders and members need to be thoughtful about the persistent barriers to collaborative communication, including differences in professional culture and training, long-standing hierarchies in health care, and team member interaction. The risk for noncollaborative patterns arising also heightens the importance of regular team meetings where the team is encouraged and held accountable for team goals by discussing the quality of communication and any other concerns. Team members need to give each other constructive feedback, provide suggestions for improvement, and discuss any disagreements or conflicts that have developed.

Review of communication and other team processes can enhance team effectiveness and ultimately patient outcomes. Effective teams "utilize feedback about team processes and productivity to make improvements in how they are functioning" (Wheelan 2013, p. 64), and research on health care teams indicates that perceived team effectiveness is "significantly and positively associated with both the number and depth of changes made to improve the quality of care for patients with chronic illness" (Shortell et al. 2004, p. 1044). Furthermore, teams that view themselves as effective take more actions to improve care (Shortell et al. 2004). These findings underscore the importance of structured time for the team to assess what's working as well as how they can improve.

Huddle

The huddle is an important practice transformation tool for creating a team approach to care (see Chapter 4, "Behavioral Health Provider Essentials," and Chapter 5, "The Primary Care Provider," for descriptions of how different team members use huddles). The huddle is a brief meeting, generally 10–15 minutes, with some teams using 30 minutes. The huddle is held each day and sometimes twice a day; most teams use the huddle to start the day, although others prefer to end their day with the huddle, reviewing the day's progress and planning for the next.

Most importantly, the huddle is a time to review the schedule for the day, identify patients who need to be seen by multiple team members or seen by team members together, and discuss workflow or team coverage concerns (see Box 3–5). The huddle provides the essential time each day for the team to plan how it will provide team-based care for the day and ensure that patients are going to receive whole person care.

Box 3–5. Checklist for Standard 10-Minute Huddle

✓ Start with review of the previous day to see if there are any unfinished follow-ups.

✓ Review status of clinic operations—staffing today, any equipment or computer problems, any special events or meetings happening today, any cancellations or open slots.

✓ Review patients on schedule with chronic conditions that need specific interventions.

✓ Review patients recently hospitalized or in emergency department.

✓ Note canceled appointments and identify backfill opportunities.

✓ Identify patients for BHP intervention or rescreening with the Patient Health Questionnaire–9 or other tool.

✓ Identify workflow challenges that need to be addressed.

Additional Elements Based on Clinic Design

✓ Case presentation of new patients.

✓ Communication or process adaptations needed.

✓ Review of registry for individuals on the schedule for the day.

✓ Review of outcome data for patients being seen that day.

✓ Diagnostic or case discussion for specific patients.

The best huddles are customized for the needs of the team and organization. The specific elements of the huddle vary from place to place, with some teams having a short session with a team lead and others using the huddle for more detailed discussion and no team leader. The effective models have a few key similarities:

1. They are targeted and have a standing agenda.
2. They occur daily.
3. The entire team attends (this is truly essential), including the BHP.
4. There is a commitment to the huddle from the team and organization.
5. Problems in the huddle are amended to make the meeting valued.
6. Huddles are included within the standard schedule for the day (often the first appointment slot).

Many teams find that early in team development, it can be useful to watch YouTube videos of huddles to get a feel for them while others engage in active practice of the huddle structure. Practicing the huddle can improve the effectiveness and the efficiency of the time scheduled and allow the team to identify the essential goals of the huddle. For one group, the behavioral health staff needed a lot of time to practice rapid and succinct psychosocial presentations that provided the essential data in a short time frame (ultimately allowing the team to review 40 patients in 30 minutes; see Cherry Street Health Services in Lardieri et al. 2014).

Huddles are not team meetings, nor do they replace the need for team meetings. Huddles are daily communication that is focused on the immediacy of patient care and effective clinic management. Although communication concerns or other team issues may be identified in huddles (and solved if they are easy), in-depth discussion of these concerns are saved for team meetings. Additionally, thorough discussion of a patient's treatment plan or a review of team-based outcomes occurs in team meetings (see the Cambridge Health Alliance Model of Team-Based Care Implementation Guide and Toolkit, listed in Appendix 3–A, for additional differences between a huddle and a team meeting).

Many organizations have tried to make the huddle an event that occurs outside of the scheduled day (e.g., starting 15 minutes ahead of the day), essentially adding time to team members' workday. This approach generally fails because it communicates that the huddle is not valued by leadership, and it fosters resentment among providers who struggle to fit it into non-work hours. Instead, organizational leaders who champion the huddle and communicate each team members' importance in attending are more likely to reap its benefits. Organizations have found that giving the first appointment of the day to the huddle works well, and the advantages of a strong huddle outweigh the expense.

SYSTEM AND OPERATIONAL SUPPORTS

Another key component of integrated care team development is the combination of structures and supports that surround the clinical team. Essentially, this is the extended organizational team that supports the delivery of care and provides the crucial tools to providers that allow them to easily collaborate and fulfill their roles. There are a number of tasks for the organizational team members that span clinical supports, technological supports, billing, and quality improvement (see Appendix 3–A for a list of resources for teams).

The clinical and technological supports generally go hand in hand and include creating clinical supports within the electronic health record. Crucial for effective collaborative care teams is the creation of a registry to track identified health metrics, a method for sharing documentation, and development of a shared treatment plan. Some organizations also provide decision supports in the electronic health record, as well as the psychiatric consultant's treatment algorithms. Other technologies that can support team communication include instant messaging, alerts, and other messaging functions that allow the team members to communicate information electronically and separately from e-mail.

Accurate and adequate billing and coding of clinical services are complex and time-intensive tasks for the organizational team members. Too often, organizations underestimate the degree to which systems and operational staff will be involved in the development and long-term support of collaborative care. The billing personnel play a crucial role by providing protocols and tools for billing, and in the best models allow providers a consistent method for billing regardless of insurer, handling the large array of specific insurance needs. This kind of significant support allows the clinical team members to improve workflow and efficiency and reduces confusion and mistakes.

As outlined in the next section, "Outcomes" (and in the appendix, "Performance and Outcome Measures for Integrated Care"), effective collaborative care is grounded in data to inform practice. Teams require data and quality improvement efforts to learn and improve the collaborative care approach in order to meet agreed-upon population goals. Research clearly demonstrates that quality improvement enhances team effectiveness (Lemieux-Charles and McGuire 2006), and yet quality improvement requires a lot of support and focused attention from extended team members. These organizational members capture the data and information that give the team evidence on lessons, mistakes, and processes in a way that improves organizational learning and ensures that failed efforts are not repeated because of loss of personnel and thereby institutional memory. For many organizations, a formal process such as the Plan-Do-Study-Act cycle (www.apiweb.org) can be instrumental in rapid improvement, although the process requires additional team member support and attention. Similarly, organizational team members codify important ingredients of care in the policies and procedures for the organization and ensure that ethics, standards of care, and regulatory, legal, and credentialing requirements are met in the team's processes (O'Daniel and Rosenstein 2008).

OUTCOMES

A core principle of the CoCM is that care is measurement based (see Chapter 1). Additionally, there is increasing evidence that measurement-based care improves patient outcomes and is better than care that does not use measurement to assess progress (Guo et al. 2015). Effective teams spend time during formal team development defining and agreeing on measurable shared outcomes: both team process outcomes and patient and population outcomes. Teams need these metrics to provide feedback on the team's success in achieving the agreed-upon goals, as well as to assess team functioning and need for refinement (Mitchell et al. 2012). The broader importance of measurement and evaluation is covered more thoroughly in the appendix, "Performance and Outcome Measures for Integrated Care"; however, what is important to note here is the role of the integrated care team in developing and reviewing specific outcomes.

Health care teams today are accountable to numerous metrics required by different systemic entities (e.g., National Committee for Quality Assurance, The Joint Commission, Primary Care Medical Home, accountable care and managed care organizations). Although these overarching structures inform outcomes for a team, each team will have unique outcomes tailored to the specific population targeted. These outcomes often include metrics regarding reduction in measurable depression, anxiety, substance use, hemoglobin A_{1c}, blood pressure, and other chronic health markers. Another common health outcome category is utilization (e.g., reduction in emergency department use, reduction in readmission to inpatient care [both psychiatric and medical], reduction in pharmacy utilization, improved follow-up with primary care scheduled visits, reduction in referral to psychiatry). Naturally, these measures may meet multiple goals (accreditation standards and collaborative care review), but the important message is that the team agrees to outcomes for the model and to treat to target for the specific population.

Generally, behavioral health screening scores and a core set of chronic medical metrics (e.g., hemoglobin A_{1c}, blood pressure) are tracked in the registry. The BHP (or care manager) then culls these data to identify, for example, those patients who are not improving or who can step down to fewer contacts (see the Chapter 4 section, "Data Management").

Patient and provider satisfaction are other important outcome measures for improving patient care and retaining providers. Both patient satisfaction and health-related quality of life (as measured by HR-QoL; Lemieux-Charles and McGuire 2006) and provider satisfaction (Levine et al. 2005) have been found to be higher when care is team based and collaborative. Provider satisfaction is also an important bottom-line consideration as providers working on high-functioning teams have greater retention (Borrill et al. 1999).

Collaborative care teams need to develop outcome goals and review data regularly to assess effectiveness. A core notion of the model is that if treatment is not working, teams adapt their overall approach to ensure patient improvement (e.g., adding additional psychiatric consultation time). It is important for teams to spend time during formal team development creating clarity about specific outcomes that they expect and agree to for the population that will be served (e.g., define their targets for treat to target). Once the team has identified these specific metrics, they also need to determine which short-term measures will be included in the registry and which long-term metrics will be reviewed as part of the team's outcomes. The more long-term or population health metrics may be reviewed in team meetings monthly or quarterly to provide feedback to the team on goal attainment and identify areas that remain a challenge. These outcomes may also inform treatment planning for specific individuals as well as overall changes to the team's approach for specific needs, such as patient engagement, coordination of services, or improved training on self-management techniques for certain illnesses. In addition to the patient outcomes, process outcomes help the team evaluate whether the delivery of care is occurring within the model design (a fidelity check of sorts) as well as assist the team in ongoing team development to enhance the team norms, processes, and overall effectiveness (see the appendix, "Performance and Outcome Measures for Integrated Care," for specific process outcomes).

CONCLUSION

At its core, development of the CoCM model is development of a team approach to care. The interaction and blending of team member knowledge and skill *is* the change in care and accounts for much of the "secret sauce" in effectiveness. The more time and resources focused on fostering a sense of *team* and formally blending culture, the more quickly and firmly the team will emerge and function. In many ways, leveraging the value of a team is a simple idea. However, organizations should not be swayed into thinking that a simple idea consequently means a simple process. Attending to the core composition and development of the team is essential for effective implementation.

REFERENCES

Bodenheimer T: Interventions to improve chronic illness care: evaluating their effectiveness. Dis Manag 6(2):63–71, 2003 14577900

Boon H, Verhoef M, O'Hara D, et al: From parallel practice to integrative health care: a conceptual framework. BMC Health Serv Res 4(1):15, 2004 15230977

Borrill C, Carletta J, Carter A, et al: The effectiveness of health care teams in the National Health Service. Aston Centre for Health Service Organization Research, Aston Business School, University of Aston, Human Communications Research Centre, Universities of Glasgow and Edinburgh, and Psychological Therapies Research Centre, University of Leeds. Commissioned by the Department of Health. 1999. Available at: http://homepages.inf.ed.ac.uk/jeanc/DOH-final-report.pdf. Accessed September 10, 2016.

Cohen DJ, Davis MM, Hall JD, et al: A Guidebook of Professional Practices for Behavioral Health and Primary Care Integration: Observations From Exemplary Sites. Rockville, MD, Agency for Healthcare Research and Quality, 2015

Coulter A, Collins A: Making shared decision-making a reality: no decision about me, without me. TheKingsFund and Foundation for Informed Medical Decision Making. 2011. Available at: http://www.kingsfund.org.uk/sites/files/kf/Making-shared-decision-making-a-reality-paper-Angela-Coulter-Alf-Collins-July 2011_0.pdf. Accessed September 19, 2016.

Cuff P: Establishing Transdisciplinary Professionalism for Improving Health Outcomes: Workshop Summary. Washington, DC, The National Academies Press, 2014, pp 1–130

Duhigg C: What Google learned from its quest to build the perfect team. The New York Times, February 25, 2016. Available at: http://www.nytimes.com/2016/02/28/magazine/what-google-learned-from-its-quest-to-build-the-perfect-team.html?_r=0. Accessed September 19, 2016.

Edmondson A: Psychological safety and learning behavior in work teams. Adm Sci Q 44(2):350–383, 1999

Guo T, Xiang YT, Xiao L, et al: Measurement-based care versus standard care for major depression: a randomized controlled trial with blind raters. Am J Psychiatry 172(10):1004–1013, 2015 26315978

Interprofessional Education Collaborative Expert Panel: Core competencies for interprofessional collaborative practice: report of an expert panel. Washington, DC, Interprofessional Education Collaborative. 2011. Available at: http://www.aacn.nche.edu/education-resources/ipecreport.pdf. Accessed September 19, 2016.

Katon W, Russo J, Lin EH, et al: Cost-effectiveness of a multicondition collaborative care intervention: a randomized controlled trial. Arch Gen Psychiatry 69(5):506–514, 2012 22566583

Kinman CR, Gilchrist EC, Payne-Murphy JC, et al: Provider-and practice-level competencies for integrated behavioral health in primary care: a literature review. (Prepared by Westat under Contract No. HHSA 290–2009–00023I). Rockville, MD, Agency for Healthcare Research and Quality, 2015

Lardieri MR, Lasky GB, Raney L: Essential elements of effective integrated primary care and behavioral health teams. SAMHSA-HRSA Center for Integrated Health Solutions. 2014. Available at: http://www.integration.samhsa.gov/workforce/team-members/Essential_Elements_of_an_Integrated_Team.pdf. Accessed September 19, 2016.

Lemieux-Charles L, McGuire WL: What do we know about health care team effectiveness? A review of the literature. Med Care Res Rev 63(3):263–300, 2006 16651394

Levi D: Group Dynamics for Teams, 5th Edition. Thousand Oaks, CA, Sage Publications, 2017, pp 1–83

Levine S, Unutzer J, Yip JY, et al: Physicians' satisfaction with a collaborative disease management program for late-life depression in primary care. Gen Hosp Psychiatry 27(6):383–391, 2005 16271652

Melek S, Norris DT, Paulus J: Economic Impact of Integrated Medical-Behavioral Healthcare: Implications for Psychiatry. Chicago, IL, Milliman, 2012

Mickan SM, Rodger SA: Effective health care teams: a model of six characteristics developed from shared perceptions. J Interprof Care 19(4):358–370, 2005 16076597

Missouri Department of Mental Health and MO Health Net: Progress Report: Missouri CMHC Healthcare Homes. 2013. Available at: https://dmh.mo.gov/docs/mentalillness/prnov13.pdf. Accessed September 19, 2016.

Mitchell P, Wynia M, Golden R, et al: Core principles and values of effective team-based health care. Discussion Paper, Institute of Medicine, October 2012. Available at: https://www.nationalahec.org/pdfs/vsrt-team-based-care-principles-values.pdf. Accessed September 19, 2016.

Nembhard IM, Edmondson AC: Making it safe: The effects of leader inclusiveness and professional status on psychological safety and improvement efforts in health care teams. J Organ Behav 27:941–966, 2006

O'Daniel M, Rosenstein AH: Professional communication and team collaboration. Agency for Health Care Research and Quality (AHRQ) Patient Safety and Quality: An evidence-based handbook for nurses. 2008. Available at: http://archive.ahrq.gov/professionals/clinicians-providers/resources/nursing/resources/nurseshdbk/index.html. Accessed September 19, 2016.

Peek CJ, National Integration Academy Council: Lexicon for behavioral health and primary care integration: concepts and definitions developed by expert consensus (AHRQ Publ No 13-IP001-EF). Rockville, MD, Agency for Healthcare Research and Quality. 2013. Available at: https://integrationacademy.ahrq.gov/sites/default/files/Lexicon.pdf. Accessed September 19, 2016.

Raney L: Integrated Care: Working at the Interface of Primary Care and Behavioral Health. Arlington, VA, American Psychiatric Publishing, 2015

Reiss-Brennan B, Brunisholz KD, Dredge C, et al: Association of integrated team-based care with health care quality, utilization, and cost. JAMA 316(8):826–834, 2016 27552616

Shortell SM, Marsteller JA, Lin M, et al: The role of perceived team effectiveness in improving chronic illness care. Med Care 42(11):1040–1048, 2004 15586830

Valentine MA, Edmondson AC: Team scaffolds: how meso-level structures support role-based coordination in temporary groups (Working Paper 12-062). Harvard Business School, 2014. Available at: http://www.hbs.edu/faculty/Publication%20Files/12-062_55befe5d-9ecd-4b42-974f-2b5c026e4769.pdf. Accessed September 19, 2016.

Wheelan SA: Creating Effective Teams: A Guide for Members and Leaders, 4th Edition. Thousand Oaks, CA, Sage Publications, 2013, pp 1–15, 44–55, 58–91

Whitebird RR, Solberg LI, Jaeckels NA, et al: Effective implementation of collaborative care for depression: what is needed? Am J Manag Care 20(9):699–707, 2014 25365745

Wynia MK, Von Kohorn I, Mitchell PH: Challenges at the intersection of team-based and patient-centered health care: insights from an IOM working group. JAMA 308(13):1327–1328, 2012 23032546

APPENDIX 3–A

Team Development Resources

Agency for Healthcare Research and Quality: TeamSTEPPS: Team Strategies and Tools to Enhance Performance and Patient Safety. Available at: www.ahrq.gov/professionals/education/curriculum-tools/teamstepps/index.html

Agency for Healthcare Research and Quality: A Guidebook of Professional Practices for Behavioral Health and Primary Care Integration: Observations From Exemplary Sites. Available at: https://integrationacademy.ahrq.gov/sites/default/files/AHRQ_AcademyGuidebook.pdf

AIMS Center: TEAMcare Implementation Guide. Available at: https://aims.uw.edu/collaborative-care/implementation-guide

Cambridge Health Alliance Model of Team-Based Care Implementation Guide and Toolkit. Available at: www.integration.samhsa.gov/workforce/team-members/Cambridge_Health_Alliance_Team-Based_Care_Toolkit.pdf

Mitchell P, Wynia M, Golden R et al: Core principles and values of effective team-based healthcare. Discussion Paper, Institute of Medicine, Washington, DC, 2012

For a review of team measurement tools, see Valentine MA, Ingrid M, Nembhard IM, et al: Measuring teamwork in health care settings: a review of survey instruments. Med Care 53(4):e16–e30, 2015

Part II

The Provider Role:
Changing Practice

CHAPTER 4

Behavioral Health Provider Essentials

Clare Scott, L.C.S.W.

Consuelo Elizabeth Mendez-Shannon, M.S.W., Ph.D.

The Core Principles of Effective Integrated Care noted in Chapter 1, "Elements of Effective Design and Implementation," start with the development of a patient-centered care team that includes at a minimum the primary care provider (PCP), a consulting psychiatric provider, and the behavioral health provider (BHP). The BHP plays a unique role on the team by bringing behavioral health skills and interventions into the exam room and to the patient. Whitebird et al. (2014) underscored the importance of this role when they discovered that the key elements of effective implementation of collaborative care include the following: "the more well defined and implemented the care manager role (BHP) the higher the rate of patient activation" and that "the care manager is seen as the right person for this job and works well in the clinic setting" (p. 2).

In the primary care setting, the BHP usually is a licensed clinical master's- or doctoral-level professional who is trained in social work or psychology, or is a licensed professional counselor or marriage and family therapist. In some settings this can be a nurse with behavioral health training, and it is becoming increasingly common to have traditional medical care managers receive additional training in behavioral health to be "integrated care managers." The terms *behavioral health provider* and *behavioral health consultant* as well as *behavioral care manager* can be used interchangeably; they frequently refer to a team member performing the same functions (behavioral health consultant is typically used in the Primary Care Behavioral Health model, referred to in Chapter 1). In addition, a shared care manager, functioning as a paraprofessional at a lower level of licensure, can perform some of the tasks of the BHP and may be included in this designation (see the section "Task Sharing or Shared Care Manager" later in this chapter). In this chapter, the abbreviation BHP will be used and can refer to any of these other titles, and several of the functions described below overlap both the Collaborative Care Model (CoCM) and Primary Care Behavioral Health model, representing a "blended" approach.

FIVE CORE FUNCTIONS

The inclusion of the BHP on a care team provides the capacity to address patient symptoms by using a holistic integrated approach and is a central feature of the CoCM. The BHP role incorporates five broad functions: patient engagement, assessment and triage, treatment intervention, follow-up and referral coordination, and data management.

Patient Engagement

Central to the historical philosophy of care and the research base for behavioral health treatment is the emphasis on the therapeutic alliance: the partnership created between therapist and client. History has taught us that unless there is a patient-provider relationship, treatment is ineffective. Duncan et al. (2010) identified relationship as the overriding common factor in effective psychotherapy. In primary care, the process of engagement or connection is also vital and must be established quickly in the fast pace of the primary care setting. The transfer of care from a PCP to a BHP, often referred to as a *warm handoff*, begins to create a shared relationship by extension of the PCP's established relationship with the patient, which allows for more rapid rapport building for the BHP. At the same time, as a result of specific training in building rapport and greater comfort with tools such as motivational interviewing, the BHP can often quicken or enhance the care team's relationship with new and existing patients. This is in essence a foundational role for the BHP: to engage patients as part of the care team and to activate them in participating in their health care. The relationship becomes strengthened when patients perceive they are being listened to and the BHP shines a light on their primary concern, which may or may not necessarily be the PCP's chief concern. The BHP helps to focus the team on the patient's goals as a top priority.

Successfully engaging patients is an essential task in effective implementation of collaborative care. As Bao et al. (2016) demonstrated, patients receiving one or more contacts with the BHP in the first month more quickly achieved clinically significant improvement than patients who did not have BHP follow-up contact within this crucial time frame (Figure 4–1). In addi-

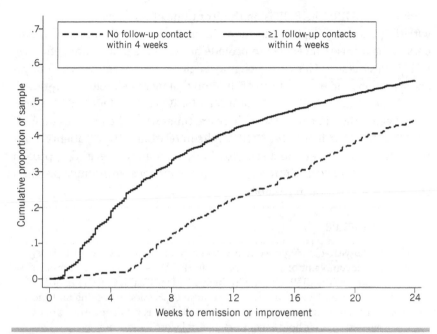

FIGURE 4–1. Time to improvement in patient response.

Note. Time to first clinically significant improvement in depression among patients in a collaborative care model, by follow-up contact in the first 4 weeks.

Source. Reprinted from Bao Y, Druss BG, Jung HY, et al.: "Unpacking Collaborative Care for Depression: Examining Two Essential Tasks for Implementation." *Psychiatric Services* 67(4):418–424, 2016. Copyright © American Psychiatric Association 2016. Used with permission.

tion, there is emerging evidence that an "e-handoff" to an off-site BHP is also acceptable to patients and is as effective as a warm handoff; the e-handoff can be an excellent alternative in a remote area or other settings (Fortney et al. 2013).

Often the BHP's engagement with the individual occurs as a result of an unplanned event. Typically, patients have scheduled an appointment with their medical provider, and in the course of the medical visit, the PCP recognizes that there is a behavioral health need through clinical assessment, patient report, or a positive behavioral health screening. It may also be that the BHP believes the individual can benefit from additional education or self-management coaching for a chronic health need or health risk (e.g., smoking). Once the concern is identified, the PCP efficiently and effectively initiates a warm handoff by communicating with the patient about the need for additional expertise from another member of the care team (see Chapter 5, "The Primary Care Provider," for examples of scripts the PCP can use to introduce the BHP). The PCP is on the front line of the engagement process with the patient and explains that as an integrated care team, different members of the team are leveraged to provide holistic care that is more effective in a given situation. This approach may begin with an examination of physical symptoms and move into an evaluation that includes mental, emotional, social, and sometimes spiritual components. When an integrated care program begins, the BHP may notice there are times when the PCP's manner of introducing the patient to the BHP results in resistance from patients. Pulling the PCP aside later and discussing ideas for a more engaging approach can help shape the PCP's introduction. The following case example provides an illustration of a warm handoff.

Case Example

HM is a 55-year-old single woman who has had numerous medical visits, with a chief complaint of stomach pain. Her PCP has ruled out any physical causes and asks the BHP to visit with her. A Patient Health Questionnaire–9 (PHQ-9) is administered as part of a routine depression screening and the score is 12. The PCP explains to the patient that she is very concerned about her pain, understands how uncomfortable and worried she must be, and tells her she is going to invite the team's BHP to meet with her to help. She does this by saying "I'm very concerned about how uncomfortable you continue to be, and I feel we need help with addressing this problem. I'm going to bring in our BHP, Joan, to talk with you." This quick and empathetic handoff brings the BHP into the exam room, and the PCP is then able to exit the room and move to the next patient.

In this case example, the provider makes the statement "I'm going to bring in our BHP…." This statement sets off a quick series of actions that may involve paging the BHP, sending the medical assistant to find the BHP, or using a flagging system to indicate which exam room requires the services of the BHP. Given this rapid series of interruptions and hallway conversations, the BHP may be asked to meet a new patient with very little information, except for knowing that there is a need for his or her services. The PCP will briefly describe the concerns to the BHP, ideally introduce the patient directly (the warm handoff), or notify the patient that the BHP is coming if the PCP wants to leave the room and move on to the next patient. Thus the BHP's role is built on flexibility, rapid and brief intervention, and the ability to balance numerous spontaneous requests with preestablished team plans (e.g., scheduled appointments or planned BHP interventions during the morning huddle; see Table 4–1 for strategies that can be used by the BHP to engage patients).

Once the BHP enters the room, intervention begins with asking the patient what his or her understanding is of why the PCP has included the BHP in the visit. This question often elicits some of the best information a patient

---

TABLE 4–1. Considerations for the BHP when entering the exam room

---

Respect dignity; wait for the patient to dress.

Greet the patient warmly.

Invite the patient to move from the exam table to a chair.

Introduce yourself; call the patient by name (if appropriate, use Mr., Ms., or Mrs.).

Explain the role of the BHP (education, intervention, and support) and the concept of behavior change, as well as any need for behavioral health services.

Keep the patient informed; let him or her know what to expect and how team-based care may differ from traditional primary care.

Acknowledge feelings, validate experiences, and acknowledge the patient's competence.

Allow the patient to fully describe his or her most concerning *immediate* problem. This may differ from the problem described by the PCP but also needs to be a problem of focus in order to quickly engage with the patient.

Recap the situation: *Scaling* (i.e., asking patients to rate how much a particular problem troubles them on a scale from 1 to 10; Nelson and Thomas 2012) can be an effective way to best understand the intensity of the concern and is a good way to share the description of the problem with the PCP.

Note. BHP=behavioral health provider; PCP=primary care provider.

can provide. It also sets the patient up to be an expert on his or her problem and the BHP to be a partner in coming up with a possible solution. It is not unusual for a patient to say, "My provider thinks my stomachache is the problem, but it is really that..." or "My doctor thinks that I am depressed, but I'm really...." This is not to say that the patient's stomach doesn't hurt or that there is no coexisting depression, but it opens the door for patients to tell the BHP *their* assessment of the issue and often the underpinnings of the problem. Thus the beginning of a conversation about how the patient can be helped is about the present situation, resources the patient may have, and small steps toward improvement he or she can take before or after leaving the exam room. In the course of the conversation the BHP is engaging, assessing the patient's emotional state, asking questions about the history of the problem, and bringing the focus of the conversation to potential inter-ventions that fit the patient's life, culture, pocketbook, and capacity.

Assessment and Triage

Assessment of the individual's mental health and substance use requires lever-aging specific diagnostic knowledge and is only part of the BHP assessment of the patient. Another essential element of understanding a patient holistically is the evaluation of how the social determinants of health play a part in a pa-tient's life. The Centers for Disease Control and Prevention (www.cdc.gov/socialdeterminants) defines these *social determinants* as

> The complex, integrated, and overlapping social structures and economic sys-tems that are responsible for most health inequities. These social structures and economic systems include the social environment, physical environment, health services, and structural and societal factors. (www.cdc.gov/nchhstp/socialdeterminants/definitions.html)

BHPs gather this kind of information to determine how the social fabric of the person's life and any mental health or substance use conditions are con-tributing to the patient's presentation in the exam room. It is the BHP who ensures effective integration of behavioral health, primary care, and social issues and then shares these factors with the care team to assist in a thor-ough assessment and care planning.

BHPs are also essential in helping the care team determine which patients are best served in primary care and which patients are most effectively treated in specialty mental health or substance use services, not unlike determining when a referral to specialty medical care is needed for serious physical illness. They can assist the PCP in managing a patient whose depression symptoms are not improving and who is now presenting with suicidal ideation, moving the patient up the stepped care ladder to a higher level of specialty behavioral health care. Likewise, a patient who is experiencing delusional or psychotic symptoms, who has never been symptomatic before, may be best helped if quickly triaged to specialty mental health once organic causes are ruled out. Finding which patients are in this crucial juncture for treatment of behavioral health conditions in the primary care setting is an important role for the BHP, and they need to be knowledgeable about the continuum of behavioral health services and the availability of those services in the community.

Nonurgent Assessment

A primary care behavioral health assessment significantly differs from an evaluation completed in specialty mental health. In traditional specialty behavioral health, assessment usually entails a lengthy interview (1 hour or more) and documentation including the individual's behavioral health history, previous treatment experiences and outcomes, and any psychological risk factors. Social-emotional development and history are thoroughly reviewed. In primary care, evaluations are far shorter in duration (5–10 minutes), with an emphasis on the present challenge and the goal to obtain just enough information to inform immediate interventions and care planning. Screening tools have preferably been administered before the exam begins, and PCPs often have historical information from longer-term relationships with patients that can be briefly summarized. For example, determining whether the patient is clinically depressed versus experiencing temporary situational stress informs the team's decision about a medication trial. The BHP aims to address the immediate need, with recognition that continued assessment can occur over time and that a brief initial intervention can inform the long-term assessment and care planning for the team. A main distinction for primary care teams in the initial assessment is that obtaining a complete psychological and psychiatric history is not necessary for the team to develop an effective treatment plan for the immediate need; rather, integrated care involves an iterative process in which additional information can be obtained over multiple visits.

At times, PCPs want assistance from the BHP in differential diagnosis (e.g., unipolar depression vs. bipolar disorder). The ability to make rapid assessments with more complex diagnostic challenges often requires the skills of more seasoned BHPs (or seasoned clinicians who become BHPs).

BHPs engage with patients by listening to the patients' view of their problem, which can be elicited by asking, "Do you know why your provider asked me to meet with you?" or "How can I help you today?" and going from there. If more time is needed than is available, an invitation for a return appointment can be offered. The BHP serves as the facilitator for the patient by more clearly identifying and acknowledging the patient's challenge and drawing out the solutions, while providing the patient with the *how* of change in order to implement the solution.

Urgent Assessment

Every primary care clinic experiences urgent or emergent behavioral health situations that can occur with patients. The BHP becomes a critical partner in these events, which are often unscheduled patient encounters. The BHP can engage the patient rapidly, and the collaborative care team has the advantage of consultation with the psychiatric consultant and the PCP to create a team-based response. However, it is often the BHPs who facilitate a rapid intervention and/or the referral to specialty behavioral health or crisis services, because BHPs often have the necessary interagency relationships. Some primary care clinics have well-developed agreements with community mental health agencies to make referrals and transfers as seamless as possible. A situation where a patient expresses suicidal thoughts, reveals serious trauma, or requires a determination of grave disability will become a priority for the BHP. Everyone on the team who is credentialed to initiate an emergency involuntary mental health hold must also be familiar with the local statutes and processes. It is often the BHP who can be the most responsive to the situation and who can rapidly engage the appropriate level of the continuum of care. BHPs are also important for reviewing and/or developing crisis protocols for their teams in the primary care clinic, setting the stage for a more focused and predictable set of procedures in an emergency.

Treatment Intervention

A valuable attribute of primary care is the long-term nature of the relationship between health care providers and patients. This series of interactions serves to maintain and enhance the relationship, even if the goal becomes very simple and small. For example, limited time in a session permits only a shared agreement between patient and provider that the patient *will* return. When the care team embraces this notion of process and time rather than specific events, it reduces the pressure to accomplish every step of an assessment, diagnosis, referral to resources, and/or a treatment plan in one visit. The key to accomplishing that goal is careful listening to what the patient is asking for help with and understanding that *the patient's* agenda for the visit is a priority.

Stepped Care

Interventions in collaborative care follow a process known as stepped care (see Chapter 1), which is an essential approach for the BHP. Each step is determined by a patient's response to treatment as indicated by assessment and data, as well as the treatment team's awareness of the treatment target. Everyone from the patient to the other care team members become part of the stepped care approach, and an increasing amount of resources in the clinic, or in collaboration with partner resources, helps patients move to their treatment target and recovery.

A patient may not move to the most appropriate step of care for a variety of reasons, including any of the following: barriers to obtaining specialty care, not being ready for change, concerns regarding privacy, cultural preferences, and so forth. The treatment team must continue providing the services that best fit primary care and avoid trying to make up for unavailable services.

Helping patients understand how systems work, enduring or persevering through the process, and continuing to support patients until they are ready for the next step is an art BHPs must perfect. Often the team member with the best relationship, or whom the patient perceives as having the right expertise, can be successful in recommending a change to a higher level of services.

Evidence-Based Brief Interventions

In primary medical clinics, it is imperative that BHPs use interventions that reflect the clinic culture, structure, and workflow related to the time allotted for them to partner with patients in their care. Therefore, BHPs use interventions that are brief, as well as evidence-based behavioral modalities that teach emotional regulation and communication skills, while educating patients about their condition. Each of these clinical interventions has a wide range of clinical applications to different populations and problems. A BHP practicing in primary care often must employ a generalist approach, in which the practitioner works with all age groups and populations, instead of working as a specialist within a specific population, diagnostic category, or therapeutic approach. Providing just the right amount of intervention needed at that appointment, staying tuned to medical necessity when there is a service that is billable, and measuring progress with validated tools are safeguards to the brevity of the intervention. Commonly used and validated treatments that should be in a BHP's toolbox include the following:

- *Motivational interviewing*: "Motivational interviewing is a directive, client-centered counseling style for eliciting behavior change by helping clients to explore and resolve ambivalence" (www.motivationalinterview.net). This conversational approach helps patients examine their ambivalence about change, with the acknowledgment by the BHP (as well as the patient) that there are both positive and negative outcomes to making change.
- *Behavioral activation*: Behavioral activation evolved from cognitive-behavioral therapy (CBT) and depression treatment. A large-scale study examining the effectiveness of therapy for serious depression found that it was the "B" in CBT that has the most effect (Dimidjian et al. 2006). This intervention examines a patient's behavior pattern, with the assumption that people who are experiencing depression are more isolative and withdrawn, and that a gradual increase in engagement of activity improves mood (Hopko et al. 2003). A study comparing CBT and behavioral activation found that behavioral activation delivered in the primary care setting by paraprofessional staff was as effective as CBT delivered by highly trained staff and presents a cost-effective solution for intervention (Richards et al. 2016).

- *Solution-focused brief therapy (SFBT)*: SFBT is a generalist approach, which assumes there are exceptions to problems and the clinician's role is to help patients discover solutions to their problems based on patients' own experiences. This approach is especially useful when there are cultural differences between the clinician and patient. A basic premise is that one small change can lead to other changes, and patients are supported in making a small change that will eventually lead them to a larger goal (Nelson and Thomas 2012). The Solution-Focused Brief Therapy Association provides a number of training tools and research information (www.sfbta.org/about_sfbt.html).
- *Problem-solving treatment (PST)*: PST is used in the Improving Mood—Promoting Access to Collaborative Treatment (IMPACT) trial to treat depression because of its validity in primary care settings. As with the other approaches listed here, it has roots in CBT but has a general goal of helping patients learn basic problem-solving skills to address their health concerns. The Advancing Integrated Mental Health Solutions Web site lists training and research support for the approach to responding to here-and-now problems (http://aims.uw.edu/impact-improving-mood-promoting-access-collaborative-treatment).
- *Mindfulness-based stress reduction*: This program was developed by Dr. Jon Kabat-Zinn as an approach to addressing a wide range of coexisting behavioral health problems and chronic diseases such as pain, HIV, cancer, and depression. It has been researched and used since 1979 and brings together mindful meditation and yoga in an evidenced-based group approach (Kabat-Zinn 1990).
- *Acceptance and Commitment Therapy (ACT)*: ACT is a therapy that differs from CBT in that instead of challenging thoughts, it "accepts" all thoughts and uses an approach that helps patients identify personal values, meaning, and purpose. The ACT acronym describes the therapeutic approach: Accept, Choose, Take action (Hayes et al. 2011).

Case Example: Brief Intervention (Solution-Focused Brief Therapy)

BD is a 32-year-old patient who reports feeling anxious daily, which has kept her from following dietary recommendations. After introducing herself, the BHP confirmed with BD why the provider asked the BHP to come into the exam room. There was agreement on the problem: BD knew she was eating poorly to feel better, but this attempt to cope with her anxiety wasn't working and she felt bad about her weight gain. When asked to "scale" the problem with her diet, BD said she was a 2 or 3 on a 1-to-10 scale (1 being she was anxious most of the time and was eating "junk food" all day long, 10 being she was eating three regular healthy meals and was going to the library to use the Internet). The BHP looked at BD and smiled, said that was an excellent goal, and asked, "Are there any days where you are able to eat a healthy breakfast and feel relaxed?" BD answered, "Yes, on mornings when I open my back door, look outside, and take a deep breath I feel better, and, yes, those days I have a decent breakfast." This realization was a surprise to BD. The BHP sat quietly giving BD some time to think. BD broke the silence, saying she could make a plan to do that every day. They had a brief conversation about what that plan would feel like, sound like, and other particulars. They agreed on this one small change, and the BHP would check back with a phone call to see if BD was able to start every day with a moment where she stood outside her back door, took a deep breath, maybe listened for the birds, and planned a healthy breakfast. This small change was an excellent start with a solution unique to BD as a result of the BHP asking simple questions and allowing BD to be the expert on her problem and solution. When the BHP called a week later, BD reported she had stepped outside most mornings, had good breakfasts, and had been to the library to use the computer three times, adding she liked the walk home for lunch because she was exercising. BD felt she was a 7 on her 1-to-10 scale.

BHPs have the crucial role of not just seeing patients who have problems but also providing extra attention to patients who have been doing well, who have been successful addressing a behavioral health problem (Tedeschi 2004), or who have been managing a chronic disease. For example, powerful interventions can include showing curiosity about how a patient has figured out how to manage pain more effectively and have fewer missed days at work, or congratulating a mother for her attentiveness to her infant. Whenever there is time, including those positive patient encounters on a BHP's daily plan is a nice approach to patient care.

Support of a Physical Health Diagnosis

BHPs are experts in behavior change and therefore can also intervene in helping patients manage physical health conditions. Some basic knowledge of the medical issue is helpful in the process, and many BHPs report that when working in the primary care setting, interacting as a team member provides a good resource for information.

Case Example: Addressing a Physical Health Problem

A PCP mentions to the BHP that she just saw a patient with hypertension and wonders if a behavioral intervention would be helpful because the patient's blood pressure has continued to be dangerously high. The patient was just getting ready to leave the exam room when the PCP knocked on the door, asking her to stay just a bit longer to meet the BHP. The patient reluctantly agreed and the BHP knew that in order to be useful she needed to be quick, because the patient was ready to leave. She confirmed quickly with the patient the problem at hand—high blood pressure—and asked if she could make a suggestion. The patient was curious and also stated that she took her medication regularly. The BHP said that there was evidence that changing breathing when feeling stressed can help lower blood pressure, and she demonstrated diaphragmatic breathing. The patient seemed interested, and the BHP asked her if she thought that she could practice daily until it felt natural. The patient agreed to try because she didn't like taking medication as the only way to address her high blood pressure. Six weeks later, the PCP pulled the BHP aside and said that she was grateful for the help—the patient's blood pressure was lowered by 10 points.

Follow-Up and Referral Coordination

It is not unusual for the BHP to be seen as the go-to person when it comes to helping patients obtain needed external resources. Referrals can include everything from locating car seats and finding housing to managing high-risk safety situations such as child maltreatment or domestic violence. Unfortunately, it is rarely simple to obtain resources, especially in safety net clinics, because of cultural and language issues, as well as transportation and expenses for the patient. In addition, referral agencies can have unforeseen barriers, such as specific criteria for acceptance, changes in referral processes, and regulations on release of information. All care teams are being required to collaborate more with external partners to ensure quality patient care, and this increase in communication requires dedicated time and effort. Once referrals are made, it is essential for a member of the care team (often the BHP for specific referrals) to follow up in order to see if a patient completed the referral. Obtaining signed release of information forms that meet compliance specifications of both the referring organization and the receiving organization, as well as sending records, reviewing records, and adjusting plans with patients, is essential to meeting patients' needs. Calling the resource to make sure the path is clear, giving patients specific contacts at the referral agency, making referrals at a pace that matches the patient's tolerance and acceptance, and closing the loop to make sure the referral occurred are all important in this process.

Task Sharing or Shared Care Manager

The task of helping people get connected to episodic service needs is often referred to as *case management* or *care coordination*. This task requires support and active participation by someone on the care team because making a referral is rarely a seamless process. The question for the care team becomes, Which team member should fulfill this function: medical assistant, nurse, social worker, psychologist, PCP, BHP, care coordinator, community health worker, or some combination? This question is best answered by following the guiding principle of maximizing the fulfillment of the function with the least expensive staff who can effectively do the job. In addition, many of these services remain nonbillable, and reserving the time of licensed staff for potentially billable services is more cost-efficient. "Working at the top of one's license" is a common phrase used to describe this way of approaching case management tasks. Care coordination and other considerations of resource allocation represent a perfect opportunity to employ task sharing or shared care management (Table 4–2) to maximize the least expensive individuals to fulfill the function. Emerging data have demonstrated that paraprofessional staff can be very effective in these roles and should be considered to fulfill appropriates functions in areas with limited resources, such as rural communities (Pietruszewski et al. 2015). In especially complex situations, teams may discuss which team member has the best relationship and/or expertise to address the referral needs of a patient in order to ensure the best care is provided. Finally, teams need to decide whether there are legal requirements for making the referral, especially in cases involving a safety risk (e.g., making a social services report of abuse or addressing a domestic violence situation). An example of a job description for a shared care manager can be found at http://uwaims.org/sif/files/Shared%20Care%20Manager%20job%20description.pdf.

Data Management

Primary care has long used flow sheets and specific protocols to treat patients with chronic illnesses such as diabetes. A data collection tool known as a *registry* (see Chapter 5, "The Primary Care Provider," and Chapter 6, "The Psychiatric Consultant") is the primary instrument used to track patient progress toward goals (improvement or decline) across a predetermined set of metrics (e.g., blood pressure, blood sugar, depression). The registry provides data to inform care teams of timely treatment adjustments, need for more specific engagement on a specific health concern, and monitoring follow-through, as well as using aggregate data for clinic performance and delivery system purposes. BHPs are well positioned to help patients understand the data that are being collected in order to improve their health and to be a constant reminder to the care team to use data to inform treatment decisions.

The use of a registry is a necessary and crucial component of the CoCM for assessing response to treatment (see https://aims.uw.edu/resource-library/care-management-tracking-system-cmts) and becomes a driver in treatment-to-target management of specific disorders (see Chapter 1). BHPs are often responsible for managing the registry and use it as a crucial tool to track care for patients who are being treated for a variety of behavioral health conditions, including depression and anxiety. This task works best with an

TABLE 4–2. Shared behavioral health provider roles utilizing paraprofessionals

Level of skill	Tasks
Paraprofessional	Screening and repeat measurement
	Supporting engagement and follow-up
	Entering data in the registry
	Phone follow-up
	Health promotion
Paraprofessional with advanced training	Brief intervention for situational stress
	Education on changing general health and behavioral health approaches
	Assisting in care coordination
Licensed staff	Assessment for more complex behavioral health needs
	Diagnostic capabilities
	Evidence-based brief psychosocial interventions, including billable events

electronic health record that identifies patients who have specific parameters entered into the chart and that generates a report showing treatment response over time. The registry can identify patients who are due for repeated measurement of their condition (e.g., use of the PHQ-9 for depression symptoms) or patients who have reached their goals and no longer meet criteria for inclusion on the registry. Managing the registry requires the BHPs to have enough authority on the care team to ask other team members to attend to needed tasks in order to get accurate and timely information. This may include giving a patient a repeat PHQ-9 or asking that a patient be briefly delayed before leaving the clinic so the BHP can quickly assess behavioral health status.

The BHP prepares the registry for the regularly scheduled (usually weekly) caseload review with the consulting psychiatric provider. The consult between the BHP and the psychiatric provider can be done by phone or in person at the clinic and includes discussion of patients' response to treatment, differential diagnosis, lack of progress toward goals, or any medication questions raised by the PCP. The BHP often communicates any possible treatment recommendations back to the PCP or may write a note in a consultation feature of the electronic medical record.

The registry tracking and caseload review are essential elements to effective integrated care and are necessary in order to use new billing codes for the CoCM (see Chapter 8, "Financing Integrated Care," for details). Therefore, it is important for the BHPs to be familiar and comfortable with these tasks. Many existing approaches to integrated care do not implement registries or specialist review and will not be eligible for this reimbursement unless they retool the BHP workforce and add mastery of these responsibilities as core competencies. Some of the process can be completed by paraprofessional staff (such as entering PHQ-9 scores into the registry), but the BHP is the key responsible party for making sure that the registry is up-to-date and actively used every day for outreach and in-reach (see Chapter 5).

WORKFLOW: PLANNED AND UNPLANNED

The workflow of a BHP (Figure 4–2) complements the typical primary care schedule. BHPs do not share the same highly scheduled appointment day of their partner PCPs. The goal is to provide flexibility in the BHP schedule, allowing them to be free to move in and out of the PCPs' prescheduled medical appointments when needed, as well as to attend to a few scheduled follow-up appointments with specific patients from a previous assessment. The BHP schedule is a dance with a delicate balance throughout the day. When the dance works smoothly, something wonderful happens. However, stepping on toes and unpredictable bumps (e.g., a medical assistant entering the room while the BHP is assessing a newborn's mother for postpartum depression) are inevitable and should be anticipated by the team as part of the process of having a flexible and highly responsive treatment approach. Beginning each day with a team huddle gives everyone the best opportunity to contribute to the process and work together on the choreography (see Chapter 3, "Team Development and Culture," for more on huddles).

Planned Consultation

Planned consultation demands a commitment from the clinic care team, operations team, and administration. It starts with the morning huddle and the registry in hand, with some preliminary preparation by the BHP if needed. A quick review of the daily schedule helps the BHP put together his or her flexible daily schedule, or "dance card." The BHP is one member of the care team who does not have a fully booked schedule of patients to see, and instead has a staggered schedule with openings for unexpected visits and

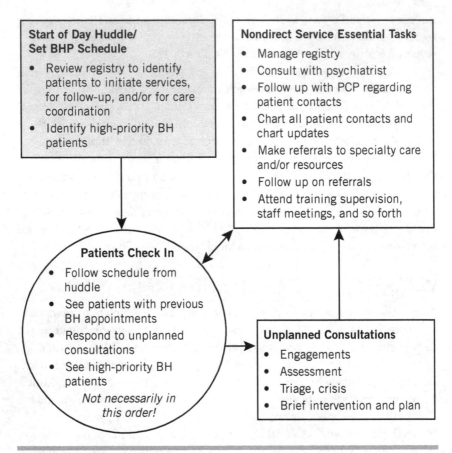

**Start of Day Huddle/
Set BHP Schedule**

- Review registry to identify
  patients to initiate services,
  for follow-up, and/or for care
  coordination
- Identify high-priority BH
  patients

Nondirect Service Essential Tasks

- Manage registry
- Consult with psychiatrist
- Follow up with PCP regarding
  patient contacts
- Chart all patient contacts and
  chart updates
- Make referrals to specialty care
  and/or resources
- Follow up on referrals
- Attend training supervision,
  staff meetings, and so forth

Patients Check In

- Follow schedule from
  huddle
- See patients with previous
  BH appointments
- Respond to unplanned
  consultations
- See high-priority BH
  patients
    *Not necessarily in
    this order!*

Unplanned Consultations

- Engagements
- Assessment
- Triage, crisis
- Brief intervention and plan

FIGURE 4–2.   BHP workflow.

Note.   BH = behavioral health; BHP = behavioral health provider; PCP = primary care
provider.

briefer 20–30 minute appointments to follow up with patients needing an
additional visit. The BHP on the team builds his or her schedule based on
who is coming in that day (Table 4–3) and then coordinates with the team to
provide ad hoc assessments as issues arise during the course of the day.

Huddles

The daily schedule for the BHP is most effectively built during the huddle
time. Patient consultations with the BHP can be "planned" in the huddle.
The team is aware that there will also be unplanned consultations that arise
throughout the day, as care team members identify patient needs that may
not have been evident from the initial patient complaint. These discoveries

TABLE 4–3. Behavioral health provider (BHP) schedule: who will I see today?

Patients...

With a scheduled BHP follow-up appointment

Who require depression follow-up, medication information, repeat Patient Health Questionnaire–9, assessment of response to treatment

Who are considered high risk, such as prenatal, recently discharged from the hospital, with complex psychosocial needs, with an uncontrolled medical condition

Who the care team has a hunch would benefit from a behavioral health assessment

are uncovered during psychosocial screenings, patient disclosure, and/or clinical observation of behavior and interactions.

Case Example: Scheduling Scenario Using the Huddle

The day begins at 8 A.M. The BHP, PCP, nurses, medical assistants, and any one who will be working that day with patients scheduled with the team meet for 20 minutes or the equivalent time period for the first appointment of the day. The BHP has accessed the daily schedule and looks at how it compares with the depression registry. There is an 8:40 A.M. patient, FR, who scheduled an appointment because of a foot injury. FR is homeless, has a history of depression, diabetes, and alcohol use. He has not been seen for more than a year and is due for a depression screen and a hemoglobin A_{1C}. The BHP puts FR on her schedule as a priority. The front desk will provide a PHQ-9 for him, and the medical assistant will collect it and enter the information into the chart after she brings him to the room. The PCP will see another patient first, which will allow the BHP to be the first provider in the room with FR, allowing her 20 minutes to start an assessment. This workflow will also allow the BHP to spend time with the PCP in the room so the team can address together with the patient how to address his presenting complaint and then review other complications with a focus on engagement to establish a stronger relationship with him and a follow-up plan.

This team has three PCPs in their group. After quickly identifying priority patients with the first PCP, the BHP moves to the other team huddles and checks in again with each PCP to identify BHP priority patients, noting patients who need follow-ups, while weaving in individually scheduled patients and additional tasks. The huddles are over at 8:20 a.m., the BHP sees her first patient at 8:30 A.M with an eye on the clock, ready to move to FR's exam room at 8:40 A.M.

Unplanned Consultation

Unplanned consultations are a part of the everyday routine and provide an important support to the PCPs and patient care. In unplanned consultation, BHPs can provide additional behavioral health resources to a chronic physical or behavioral health concern, assisting the patient in learning self-management techniques and engaging in readiness for behavior change. BHPs can also address relationship issues, parenting problems, pain management, and sleep problems as well as urgent behavioral health concerns, such as suicidal ideation. A situation may arise that requires brief intervention, triage, or crisis response, and space is left open in the BHP's schedule, anticipating the need for assessment and intervention. Sometimes information is shared in the daily huddle about patients who may end up needing unplanned consultation, but typically these sessions are unpredictable.

> **The need for flexibility and resiliency:** "No matter how much you plan your day, it may turn out completely different, so flexibility and resiliency are a must."—*Behavioral health provider*

The Daily Dance Card

At the end of the day, all planned and unplanned activities ultimately may look like the day that was forecasted at the huddle, or they may look completely different (Table 4–4). In one of the author's clinics, this fluctuating schedule was referred to as the "daily dance card," reflecting the planned nature of the day's activities, much like dance cards used in formal dances in the past that were interrupted by unplanned events. Being flexible and adaptable are important traits for the BHP to possess in managing the day's events, and it is often this unpredictable course of events that adds to the excitement many experience doing this work.

TEAM COMMUNICATION

Working With PCPs

There is an art to PCP and BHP communication, and both parties need to be invested in making it work. BHPs often need to be flexible and learn to vary their style based on the PCP personality and style of practice. For example, some PCPs just want concise "bullets" on patient history or symptoms from the BHP assessment, and other providers want greater patient

TABLE 4–4. Example of the behavioral health provider's (BHP's) dance card before and at the end of the day

Dance card after the morning huddle	Actual dance card by 5 P.M.
8:20 A.M.—Meet with patient AS and Dr. Lewis in exam room 4 to review depression treatment (PHQ-9 needed).	8:20 A.M.—Met with patient AS; called out for introduction to new patient in room 1 with Dr. Anderson.
8:40 A.M.—Open	8:40 A.M.—Dr. Anderson's patient BN has history of depression and the PHQ-9 is 20 with score of 2 on question 9 (suicidal thoughts).
9:00 A.M.—Meet with patient AA re: anxiety.	Reviewed generalized anxiety disorder, brief intervention, and follow-up plan.
	9:15 A.M.—Phone call to psychiatric consultant re: AS and BN; medication recommendations.
9:20 A.M.—Open	9:30 A.M.—Share call information from psychiatric consultant with Dr. Lewis and Dr. Anderson.
9:40 A.M.—Open	9:35 A.M.—AA did not show for 9:00 appointment; left voice message for her to call and reschedule.
	9:40 A.M.–10:00 A.M.—Phone call to follow up with referral to CMHC.

TABLE 4–4. Example of the behavioral health provider's (BHP's) dance card before and at the end of the day (*continued*)

Dance card after the morning huddle	Actual dance card by 5 P.M.
10:00 A.M.—Scheduled follow-up appointment.	10:00 A.M.–10:40 A.M.—Saw patient KL for follow-up re: depression and smoking cessation.
10:20 A.M.—In session.	
10:40 A.M.—Open	
11:00 A.M.—Follow-up with patient TR, his wife, and Dr. Lewis re: back pain.	11:00 A.M.–11:05 A.M.—Hallway discussion with PCP to discuss options for TR before entering the exam room together, including chronic pain group referral.
11:20 A.M.—Open	11:05 A.M.–11:40 A.M.—Review coping strategies with TR. Introduce group as part of treatment plan.
11:40 A.M.—Pediatric appointment with JM (7 years) and mom re: possible ADHD behavior, sign releases for school.	11:45 A.M.—Give JM's mom Conners' Rating Scales for ADHD to complete and copy for teacher; set follow-up appointment; discuss behavior at home and ideas for both JM and mom, starting with ride back to school.
12:00 P.M.—Pediatric appointment with homeless teen TS regarding cutting behavior, sign release for shelter, CMHC.	12:00 P.M.–12:20 P.M.—With establishing connection, sign release, set up follow-up.

TABLE 4–4. Example of the behavioral health provider's (BHP's) dance card before and at the end of the day *(continued)*

Dance card after the morning huddle	Actual dance card by 5 P.M.
12:20—Open	12:20 P.M.–1:00 P.M.—PHQ-9 (for adolescents) and suicide assessment with TS and safety plan. Set up follow-up and decision making for referral to higher level of service. Discuss need to collaborate with other organizations.
12:40 P.M.—Open	
1:00 P.M.–2:00 P.M.—Lunch	1:00 P.M.–1:45 P.M.—All-clinic meeting scheduled.
	1:45 P.M.–2:00 P.M.—Eat, run to bathroom.
2:10 P.M.—Initial appointment with patient BH who is experiencing breathing problems, to rule out panic disorder.	2:10 P.M.–2:20 P.M.—PCP warm handoff to patient BH with breathing problem, GAD-7 completed, reviewed relaxation techniques, set up follow-up.
2:20 P.M.—Detox referral for NW.	2:20 P.M.–3:00 P.M.—Call to detox unit for NW re: referral, charting.
3:00 P.M.—Meet with psychiatric consultant to review registry.	
3:30 P.M.–3:45 P.M.—Covisit with Dr. Anderson's patient with high hemoglobin A_{1c} per huddle schedule.	

TABLE 4–4. Example of the behavioral health provider's (BHP's) dance card before and at the end of the day (*continued*)

Dance card after the morning huddle	Actual dance card by 5 P.M.
3:40 P.M.—Open	3:45 P.M.–3:50 P.M.—Phone call to patient with follow-up regarding treatment plan started 1 week ago; left message for patient to call BHP back and leave message regarding progress.
4:00 P.M.—Open	3:50 P.M.–4:30 P.M.—See urgent patient shared with CMHC who was asking for prescription change; checked record at CMHC (has shared access and credentialing); saw patient had missed last appointment with psychiatrist; facilitated call with patient to get bridge script and rescheduled at CMHC.
4:20 P.M.—Follow-up with patient HC regarding PHQ-9 score.	4:20 P.M.–4:50 P.M.—Reviewed PHQ-9 update with patient HC, noticed improvement in score and asked patient to share what he had done to feel better.
4:40 P.M.—Open, last appointment on schedule.	4:50 P.M.–5:30 P.M.—Charting

Note.   ADHD=attention-deficit/hyperactivity disorder; CMHC=community mental health center; GAD-7=Generalized Anxiety Disorder 7-item scale; PCP=primary care provider; PHQ-9=Patient Health Questionnaire–9.

history and context. Sometimes the PCPs want to know that their concerns about the patient are being addressed to reduce their own anxiety about a troubling situation. BHP communication with PCPs can also be a central bridge between the patient and the care team by connecting the patient's stated needs and goals with the provider's assessment and priorities. Finally, patient needs may not be stated in the same language as a PCP's assessment, and the BHP has an opportunity to bridge that gap. In this process, the BHP serves as a patient translator by conveying the patient's perception of the problem to the provider and bringing the provider's concerns to the patient.

In addition, BHPs are in a position to introduce a culture shift for PCPs, because BHPs are better trained to tolerate ambiguity and variations in patients' process as they move toward healthy behavior or change. Skillful BHPs manage their own strong feelings of helplessness or similarities to their own experience (transference) with their team and with supervisor support. They can bring that same skill to PCPs who struggle with the need to rescue patients, who become frustrated with barriers to resources for deserving patients, and who have anxiety about psychosocial situations where the care team has no control. BHPs can also model professional neutrality and an approach to establishing firmer boundaries when there are more complicated patient situations, which may occur with personality or substance use disorders. The experience of watching a skilled BHP "shift into neutral" during a tense encounter can be a valuable learning opportunity for all clinic providers and help them more skillfully handle a similar situation at a later time.

Communicating with PCPs: "One BHP told me she felt like the act of giving feedback about patients to the PCPs on her team was similar to her work as a waitress. Each PCP has a different communication style, just like each table she was responsible for in the restaurant. Some customers wanted just the basic information, others wanted full explanations regarding preparation and sourcing of food."—*C.S., Colorado*

As a team develops, the BHP and PCP have more and more shared experiences from which they begin to build rapport and learn to trust each other. Both have ample time to see each other in action with patients, team members, and staff. There is a shared responsibility to create a climate where questions, feedback about the work, responses to patients, diagnosis, and problem solving when patients are not improving are welcomed. Patients see this working relationship in action, and it is the professionals in the room who set the tone for respectful and hopeful communication.

Communication With Psychiatric Consultants

Because most psychotropic medications used in the United States are prescribed in primary care, PCPs are often in need of support and consultation with psychiatric providers (Graff et al. 2010). BHPs can share the task of obtaining the psychiatric consultant's recommendation by collecting additional history, previous medication responses, and other information; BHPs can communicate this information to the consultant on behalf of the PCP. They can then communicate the recommendation to the prescribing PCP, serving as a conduit of information. One goal of psychiatric consultation in an integrated program is to increase the PCP's comfort and effectiveness with prescribing psychotropic medication, and the BHP is a valuable intermediary in this process. It is important that the BHP does not go beyond his or her scope of practice and recommend a specific medication or dosing strategy, although it may be tempting as the BHP becomes quite familiar with the psychiatric consultant's typical recommendations. In addition, there should be abundant opportunities for the PCP and consulting psychiatric providers to work together, for example, by phone or in monthly case reviews. The BHP can also assist by offering to call the psychiatric consultant for the provider, which can be particularly helpful if the PCP is reluctant to make the call or does not see the need for consultation as clearly as the BHP does. This may at times feel awkward if the BHP perceives that the PCP is not making the correct treatment decision, and a private conversation with the psychiatric consultant may help with troubleshooting the issue.

The relationship, collaboration, and communication between the BHP and the psychiatric consultant is a central component of the integration program. Because the BHP is on site and the first contact patients have with the behavioral health services in a primary care setting, the BHP often becomes the conduit for treatment conversations between patients, PCPs, and psychiatric consultants. Building trust through candid, supportive communication allows the BHP to leverage the psychiatric consultant's expertise. Each member of the team must have quick and easy access to each other and feel empowered to speak to any other member of the team to get clarity on a plan, confirm a diagnosis, understand subtleties of medication, and get another voice in the conversation. This is challenging work, and teams are stronger when they have respect for each other's skills and unique contributions. This is particularly important in the BHP–psychiatric consultant relationship when coordinating care in the presence of the PCP. The psychiatric consultant needs to be respectful and supportive of the BHP's assessment and recommendations and not attempt to appear more knowledgeable or try to trump the BHP's suggestions.

ADDITIONAL FUNCTIONS

Individual Therapy

BHPs do not engage in traditional psychotherapy; however, they do engage in sessions that are targeted to behavior change and self-management skills development. Therapy looks more like consultation in the primary care setting than like traditional psychotherapy because the focus is on behavior change as opposed to addressing underlying psychosocial issues. One of the key distinctions for sessions is that interruptions in primary care are inevitable during one-on-one sessions with a BHP, much as interruptions are part of the process for the PCP. Patients are accepting of this flow, especially when they are informed in advance and because they are familiar with the primary care environment. Having relevant educational handouts available for a patient to read, inviting them to reflect on the discussion taking place before the interruption, or suggesting they take a few moments during the absence of the BHP to practice a relaxation skill such as diaphragmatic breathing can be a good use of the time while waiting for the BHP to return. It is often the untrained BHP who struggles with this change because of his or her training in the importance of the uninterrupted therapy hour.

Clinics engage in various models to provide ongoing psychotherapy. A clinic may identify specific BHPs to provide consultation to primary care certain days of the week and then have other days when the BHPs provide traditional therapy (this approach can be particularly useful in pediatric populations). Or as their primary role, BHPs may refer patients to in-house specialty behavioral health staff to provide therapy. Some clinics have co-located staff from specialty mental health clinics or have streamlined referrals to the local mental health center when individual therapy is the best intervention.

Group Therapy

Primary care practices have been particularly adept at developing effective group care for certain patient populations (Dobrof et al. 1990) by using evidence-based treatment, such as the following: chronic disease self-management (Lorig et al. 2006), *Seeking Safety* (Najavits 2001), CenteringPregnancy (see www.centeringhealthcare.org/what-we-do/centering-pregnancy), pain management, and diabetes care. BHPs can facilitate, cofacilitate, and provide education as needed, which then allows an opportunity for behavioral health assessment and intervention that fits into the primary care environment. The decision clinics make in how to use behavioral health resources depends on the need and available services at the site. The best way to use limited resources is to strive to keep everyone working at the top of their license. For example, a paraprofessional or case manager can run a CenteringPregnancy group effectively, and the BHP may come in as needed to introduce topics such as partner abuse or parent-child attachment. Or a clinic may decide that including a BHP is essential for a pain management group where sessions provide training in emotional regulation, stress reduction, anxiety management, substance use, and changes related to lifestyle and social skills.

OPERATIONS

Staffing

A common question related to the integration of behavioral health care is how to determine the number of BHPs needed in a given clinic setting. The answer depends primarily on the burden of behavioral health conditions in the population of patients that have been selected for the integrated care initiative. The prevalence of behavioral health burden in a setting can be determined by using clinic data analysis for information such as the percent of patients with depression, anxiety, substance use disorders, chronic pain, or other concerns (see Chapter 1). For example, there is a marked difference in the number of BHPs that are needed in a clinic with a low burden (and less severe presentation) of behavioral health conditions, such as a clinic with mainly privately insured patients in a more affluent area, compared with a clinic serving a homeless population. The caseload for the BHP somewhere in the middle of these parameters might be 60–80 patients in their registry at a time, whereas 80–100 patients for a private clinic and 30–50 patients for a homeless population would be reasonable. It is important not to understaff the clinic because the intensity of the engagement and number of contacts likewise will be diminished. The effectiveness research informs us that if understaffing occurs, outcomes will not be achieved (see the section "Patient Engagement" earlier in this chapter). Hiring additional staff as caseloads fill, including paraprofessionals to complement the team and take on some of the tasks that can be handled at a lower level of licensure, is a possible solution to preventing overfilling of caseloads (a useful resource for staffing guidelines can be found at https://aims.uw.edu/resource-library/guidelines-care-manager-caseload-size).

Hiring

Hiring a BHP to become a member of a collaborative care team is an art form in itself and one of the most important decisions to be made. The mantra in the field, given the significance of this position on the team, is "hire the right person." Although more postgraduate training programs are including instruction in health psychology, and specifically work in integrated care, the workforce is still not at a level where licensed BHPs are readily available for all the open positions. With that reality in mind, on-the-job training while hiring for specific individual personal strengths becomes essential (Table 4–5). Most therapists are not trained in the work of a BHP and come to the job with the usual skill set obtained for traditional psychotherapy, often with a narrow population focus. This training has very little in common with the expectations of primary care and the breadth of patients and needs that are seen in a primary care setting. The BHP needs to be capable of working with a wide range of patients including young children, first-time parents, adolescents, and elders and needs to be prepared to engage in interventions averaging 20–30 minutes. However, personality style can overcome some of the training gaps. If the BHP has a personality style that lends itself to an ability to contribute to a team, has the confidence and tenacity to function as a peer with medical providers, shows a curiosity about the interface between physical and behavioral problems, and can develop an understanding of how systems work both on a macro and micro level, then appropriate orientation to the new environment of primary care may go smoothly. It is important also that the BHP be able to maintain a philosophy that patients *do* want to feel better, and when the BHP and team listen carefully, patients tell the team members how they can be helpful. As a result of the importance of personal style and characteristics, interviewing potential candidates for these characteristics is crucial (see Appendix 4–A for sample interview questions).

Cultural Competency

BHPs who understand the cultural needs of the clinic's patients will increase the efficacy of their role (see also Chapter 5). Cultural awareness and sensitivity to different populations served at the clinic is an essential first step in engaging clients. There is value in learning about the specific demographics served by the clinic so that engagement and treatment plans adhere to cultural fluency and representation. For example, a clinic primarily serving Spanish-speaking patients will benefit from a BHP who identifies with a multicultural identity and can speak a second language. Patients may be more likely to trust a professional who can converse with them in their own language, affirming the therapeutic relationship and increasing the ability to build the trust necessary for effective treatment.

Although it is valuable for patients to feel connected culturally with the BHP, it is equally important for treatment to feel culturally relevant. General information known about Mexican culture, for example, may not be relevant

TABLE 4–5. Attributes of a great behavioral health provider

Believes that brief treatment *is* effective treatment

Willing and capable to provide care to *all* age groups, infants through elders

Skilled in addressing typical presenting behavior problems in primary care, including but not limited to chronic pain, trauma, grief, relationship and parenting problems, acculturation issues, substance use, and mood and anxiety disorders

Curious about the interface between behavioral health and physical health

Convinced that patients *are* capable of change

Comfortable with efficient and quick mental health assessments

Able to triage; understands who can be helped in primary care and who needs a different level of care

Understands team dynamics and varying communication styles

Sees the work as most effective when team members are working together, not working independently

Willing to walk into a new situation with staff and patients with confidence and curiosity

Adaptable to change and uses creative thinking to addressing varying situations

Has an open nonjudgmental stance toward individuals and families

Manages personal stress well and helps monitor team stress and conflict levels

---

to those from different regions of Mexico. Knowing about the varying approaches to the medical model and wellness approach deepens how BHPs practice with patients from different cultures, even when they may be from the same country.

Across the country, clinics are experiencing challenges in filling positions with personnel who fit these criteria and meeting the cultural needs of varying patients. At a national level, there is development of specific policy initiatives, such as the standards of the Culturally and Linguistically Appropriate Services in Health and Health Care (www.thinkculturalhealth.hhs.gov/clas), as well as state and local efforts for workforce training focused on cultivating a more diverse professional workforce. There is particular momentum around adapted training and workforce development within social work, such as the Metropolitan State University of Denver's Behavioral Health Workforce Education and Training for Professionals Project grant (see www.msudenver.edu/socialwork/scholarshipsawards/hrsastipendprogram). This stipend-based program helps social work students by providing field placement stipends for a concentration year. Or students with advanced standing can be placed at agencies that provide intervention and prevention services to at-risk children, youth, and transitional age youth and/or their families, with specific attention to prevention and early intervention with high-risk activities, including violence. Because of the focus on prevention, primary care becomes an especially appropriate setting for an internship serving this population.

Training New BHPs

Much of the training of BHPs over the past 10 years has been on the job because course work such as that mentioned above has not been readily available or affordable. Primary care organizations have partnered with community mental health centers to bring in trained BHPs, some of whom embraced the model and others who questioned its effectiveness and turned out to be a poor fit for the clinic. Other primary care sites have developed their own training program guided by workshops, literature, Web sites, learning collaboratives, and consultants. There has been a great deal of frustration that social workers, psychologists, and professionals in related fields have not had academic training to support integrated care. Several programs have taken on the challenge and are leading the way by offering certificates, scholarships, and standardized training, such as the following:

- Free online self-study modules are available (including a certificate for completion) from the University of Washington Advancing Integrated Mental Health Solutions Center (https://aims.uw.edu/collaborative-care/team-structure/care-manager).
- An online classroom for new and experienced social workers and others includes interactive group assignments at the University of Michigan School of Social Work (http://ssw.umich.edu/programs/msw/financial-aid/integrated-health-scholarship-program).
- An online introductory overview for BHPs new to integrated care is offered at the University of Massachusetts Center for Integrated Primary Care (www.umassmed.edu/cipc).

Each program has its own strengths and should be assessed for how it works in a particular setting and budget.

Shadowing as a Teaching Technique

There are numerous approaches to training for the BHP role beyond learning brief interventions and disease-related information. Training a BHP to understand clinic culture, teamwork, and workflow is essential to creating a successful BHP. Shadowing has emerged as a very useful strategy for orienting and training. This approach is most useful when a new BHP is joining the team and there are seasoned staff on-site. Care teams require the BHP to use skills to engage, build trust, triage, and work collaboratively. The Shadow Tool (Scott et al. 2013) incorporates a list of tasks to help the newly hired BHP learn the nuances of working in the primary care setting and to develop effective communication skills while being observed by a trainer. The hallmark of the Shadow Tool is its focus on specific, observable behaviors the trainee can see while shadowing an experienced BHP in a primary care clinic. The trainee is then observed doing the task, and proficiency can be evaluated. This tool can be an effective means of introducing a new employee to the position, collaborative care in general, workflows, team dynamics, and population-based care. The tool provides guidance for exactly what a new BHP should be looking for when observing an experienced BHP in practice and an opportunity to discuss what was observed in order to understand the motives and reasons for specific behaviors.

Triage

Understanding how to triage patient needs and knowing a BHP's role based on clinic priorities will go a long way toward helping BHPs prioritize treatment decisions, especially during unscheduled patient encounters and provider situations that spontaneously occur during the day. A BHP will need to manage competing priorities and have the team's support as they move through the day with diverse scenarios, such as being asked to see an adolescent with suicidal ideation in exam room 1 while the patient in exam room 2 is due for a PHQ-9 and follow-up with a registry entry. It is important for the team to build a level of trust with the BHP so that conflicts do not arise when the BHP delays going to exam room 2 when exam room 1 takes priority.

Documentation

It is important that the BHP's notes are fully visible and accessible to the entire team and not hidden behind a firewall in the interest of "privacy" or a misinterpretation of the Health Insurance Portability and Accountability Act. BHPs are not always trained to chart in a medical record and struggle with what should be included or left out. Limiting charting to "what is necessary" including describing the event, substantiating a diagnosis, and documenting the plan can serve as a guide. Learning to chart in this manner means learning to leave out language that gives specifics about trauma, details that identify family members, and what serves as the BHP's memory of the situation. There is an art to charting, but once mastered, worries about sharing information are relieved; charting becomes efficient and includes data that helps the care team support patient goals, track progress, and coordinate care. Also, unless BHPs are providing "psychotherapy" and keeping psychotherapy notes, which are kept separate from the medical chart, privacy issues are usually not a problem (McGraw et al. 2015). Most integrated programs that provide therapeutic interventions discourage keeping "psychotherapy notes" because of liability concerns. A reasonable place to start with charting decisions involves support from quality improvement and billing departments. Each event code or billing code has specific criteria for that event. To chart most efficiently, every clinician needs to be familiar with the charting requirements for the codes they use. For example, a brief assessment has different charting requirements than individual therapy.

Scheduling and Building the BHP Template

The role of the BHP is a new one at many sites, and there are few established measures of job performance at this time (see the appendix, "Performance and Outcome Measures for Integrated Care"). It is also a role that is being developed as patient outcomes are becoming part of job performance indicators, rather than simply relying on productivity or other metrics. Medical systems that are looking to improve the care of patients with mental health and substance use disorders should be wary of spending time and money to simply co-locate mental health specialists within primary care. Typically, BHPs do not, nor should they, have a back-to-back schedule of 20–30 minute appointments filled by a central scheduling process, nor should they have back-to-back 50-minute traditional therapy slots they have filled at their own discretion (co-location). An ideal arrangement is a schedule with blocks of openings that are prefilled during the morning huddle based on patient, provider, and chronic care guidelines intermingled with open slots for unplanned events.

When BHPs are first placed in primary care clinics, there may be a lack of understanding of how to use their skills, and they may be underutilized initially. Many strategies can help the staff begin to employ the skills of BHPs, including having BHPs shadow the PCP for a day without any interventions, and then summarize for the PCP what they observed and how they may have been helpful with different patients. The entire care team has the responsibility to use behavioral resources effectively and efficiently, but because the newest role on the team is the BHP, it becomes the BHP's specific charge to help the team understand and incorporate his or her role into patient care.

Table 4–6 provides a list of strategies the BHP can use to increase BHP utilization and team work.

The importance of being part of the team: "It does not matter how excellent your clinical skills are if you are not seen as part of the team and the medical providers do not see you as beneficial to their patients and their work."—*Behavioral health provider*

Supervision

Many practices have set up integrated programs via contractual or leased agreements between medical and behavioral health organizations, in which an employee of one organization is embedded in another. This arrangement adds to the complexity of employee management and can be dealt with through agreements by leadership of the separate organizations. However, given the speed and unpredictable nature of the work, it is important for everyone's peace of mind to know who the supervisor is for each employee. This should be determined in advance so the embedded BHP knows whom to contact for administrative decisions (e.g., for paid time off, an increase in pay) and for clinical decisions (e.g., "Should I call child protection?" or "Does this person meet criteria for a mandatory mental health hold?").

Monitoring for Burnout

BHPs can sometimes become overwhelmed by the complexity of problems patients bring to the exam room. Burnout is an ongoing management problem and an opportunity for training. Many resources are available to help staff in this area, and it is often the behavioral health staff who have the sophisticated antennae to notice burnout trends on a team. Providing an opportunity for behavioral health team members to bring burnout concerns to the attention of clinic management can be helpful. It is also an area where the culture of behavioral health differs from physical health. An ongoing practice in the field of therapy is to provide clinical supervision even after licensure. Because the basic tools of the trade are language and relationships, it is not unusual for behavioral health clinicians to get their own personal experience confused with a patient's situation or to experience vicarious trauma, for example; these and similar issues can be addressed through clinical supervision.

Another useful resource is the use of basic mindfulness techniques (Kabat-Zinn 1990). Staff can practice the very skill they are teaching their patients to

TABLE 4–6. Strategies for a behavioral health provider (BHP) to increase BHP utilization and team work

Create a culture of "yes" or a culture of availability; express pleasure at being asked to see a patient.

Teach patients that you will be interrupted and teach providers to interrupt you.

Increase your comfort with short encounters with the primary goal of making a connection with both patients and providers.

Use huddles to create a daily plan.

Help the team to see your value; for example, make handouts on a particular topic of interest or do a presentation on an issue at the provider meeting.

Count encounters to monitor progress; aim for 7–10 contacts a day at a minimum.

Count medical provider referrals for behavioral health services to see where the business is coming from (and who may need a reminder of the BHP's availability).

Shadow a primary care provider for a day, keeping a list of all the ways you could have intervened with patients, and share this with the provider at the end of the day.

manage pain and emotional dysregulation. Being present in the moment, giving full attention to the task at hand as opposed to anticipating what will be next or trying to multitask, will increase both efficiency and effectiveness. A practice of mindfulness is an effective tool to manage the inevitable stress brought on by working in a busy primary care clinic. Clearing one's mind and preparing for the next encounter is an excellent practice of mindfulness skills. BHPs must allow themselves to stop, take a deep breath, and exhale to ready themselves to be nonjudgmental and focus on the task at hand. The BHP can also guide the team in a moment of mindful meditation following the morning huddle, providing a powerful tool to help the group manage the day.

REFERENCES

Bao Y, Druss BG, Jung HY, et al: Unpacking collaborative care for depression: examining two essential tasks for implementation. Psychiatr Serv 67(4):418–424, 2016 26567934

Dobrof J, Umpierre M, Rocha L, et al: Group work in a primary care medical setting. Health Soc Work 15(1):32–37, 1990 2318462

Dimidjian S, Hollon SD, Dobson KS, et al: Randomized trial of behavioral activation, cognitive therapy, and antidepressant medication in the acute treatment of adults with major depression. J Consult Clin Psychol 74(4):658–670, 2006 16881773

Duncan B, Miller S, Wampold B, Hubble M: The Heart and Soul of Change: Delivering What Works in Therapy, 2nd Edition. Washington, DC, American Psychological Association, 2010, p 113

Fortney JC, Pyne JM, Mouden SB, et al: Practice-based versus telemedicine-based collaborative care for depression in rural federally qualified health centers: a pragmatic randomized comparative effectiveness trial. Am J Psychiatry 170(4):414–425, 2013 23429924

Graff CA, Springer P, Bitar GW, et al: A purveyor team's experience: lessons learned from implementing a behavioral health care program in primary care settings. Fam Syst Health 28(4):356–368, 2010 21299282

Hayes S, Strosahl K, Wilson K: Acceptance and Commitment Therapy. New York, Guilford, 2011

Hopko DR, Lejuez CW, Ruggiero KJ, et al: Contemporary behavioral activation treatments for depression: procedures, principles, and progress. Clin Psychol Rev 23(5):699–717, 2003 12971906

Kabat-Zinn J: Full Catastrophe Living. New York, Delacorte Press, 1990

Lorig K, Sobel D, Laurent D, et al: Living a Healthy Life With Chronic Conditions. Boulder, CO, Bull Publishing, 2006

McGraw D, Belfort R, Dworkowitz A: Fine print: rules for exchanging behavioral health information in California. California Health Care Foundation, July 2015. Available at: http://www.chcf.org/~/media/MEDIA%20LIBRARY%20Files/PDF/PDF%20F/PDF%20FinePrintExchangingBehavioral.pdf. Accessed September 20, 2016.

Najavits L: Seeking Safety. New York, Guilford, 2001

Nelson TS, Thomas FN: Handbook of Solution Focused Brief Therapy: Clinical Applications. London, Routledge, 2012

Pietruszewski PB, Mundt MP, Hadzic S, et al: Effects of staffing choices on collaborative care for depression at primary care clinics in Minnesota. Psychiatr Serv 66(1):101–103, 2015 25269565

Richards D, Ekers D, McMillan D, et al: Cost and Outcome of Behavioural Activation Versus Cognitive Behavioral Therapy for Depression (COBRA): a randomized, controlled, non-inferiority trial. Lancet 388(10047):871–880, 2016 27461440

Scott C, Mendez-Shannon CE, Peck J, et al: Training behavioral health professionals: how to join a medical team. 2013. Available at: http://www.integration.samhsa.gov/workforce/Training_Behavioral_Health_Professionals_Shadow_Tool.pdf. Accessed September 20, 2016.

Tedeschi R: Posttraumatic growth: a new perspective of psychotraumatology. Psychiatr Times 21(4):4, 2004

Whitebird RR, Solberg LI, Jaeckels NA, et al: Effective implementation of collaborative care for depression: what is needed? Am J Manag Care 20(9):699–707, 2014 25365745

APPENDIX 4–A

Interview Questions for Hiring Successful Behavioral Health Providers

1. Given the job description, briefly describe how your education and professional experience make you an excellent candidate for this position (e.g., child experience, adult experience, common problems, depression, anxiety, chronic pain, personality disorders, mood disorders, adult/child attention-deficit/hyperactivity disorder, trauma, grief, relationship and parenting problems, acculturation issues, substance use)?
2. How do you handle a clinical situation where you might not have direct training or experience?
3. When we describe the treatment used in this program as "brief," what does that mean to you? How do you think it compares with long-term treatment?
4. Please give an example of a time when you used triage skills during a mental health assessment. How would you rule out the need for a different level of behavioral health treatment than what was available at your agency or setting?
5. Please describe your experience with designing a behavioral health or self-management treatment plan developed collaboratively with a patient.
6. Please describe your experience working with medical providers and your experience working as part of a team. How would you approach a situation where your idea differs from how the primary care provider or psychiatric consultant is proposing to handle a situation with a patient?
7. Are you familiar with working in primary care clinics and how that culture may differ from the specialty behavioral health setting? Can you describe how those differences might affect your work?
8. How do you handle interruptions by other team members when you are with a patient?
9. Do you have experience with managing a registry?
10. Each of us has "hot buttons" when working with others and working in multiple systems. What is one of your "hot buttons" that you have encountered in your work and how do you handle it?
11. How do you tend to manage stress in general?
12. What do you need from a clinical supervisor to support your work?

CHAPTER 5

The Primary Care Provider

Carolyn Shepherd, M.D.

Chris Keenan, M.D., M.P.H.

Kristen Roessler, M.D., FAAP

Jack Todd Wahrenberger, M.D., M.P.H.

Julianna Reece, M.D., M.B.A., M.P.H.

OVERVIEW OF THE PRIMARY CARE LANDSCAPE

Primary care is changing. The provider-centered practice where all decisions and orders are initiated by doctors will cease to exist because it does not and cannot reach the quadruple aim of improving health outcomes, improving patient and provider experience of care, and reducing costs (Bodenheimer and Sinsky 2014). For over 60 years, primary care has been "testing" the current volume-driven model, which has produced relatively small health improvements and has increased per capita cost of care. Health care costs are high, national clinical outcomes are at best mediocre, and providers are leaving the profession in frustration—and there are not enough trainees in the pipeline to make up the losses. If primary care is to be successful, it must look significantly different. The current trend is toward team-based care to improve health care delivery (Table 5–1) (Bodenheimer et al. 2014).

Transformative changes in health care delivery described in this book include adding behavioral health providers (BHPs) and psychiatric consultants as members of primary care teams. Patients in these practices experience the benefit of timely handoffs from primary care provider (PCP) to BHP, as well as behavioral health interventions for common issues, such as depression, anxiety, and substance use disorders, and without significant delays in patient flow through the practice. The successful primary care model of the future that improves the health of the population it serves will integrate BHPs,

TABLE 5–1. The 10 essential building blocks of high-performing primary care

Foundational elements

1. Engaged leadership

2. Data-driven improvement

3. Empanelment

4. Team-based care

Building blocks supported by the foundational elements

5. Patient-team partnership

6. Population management

7. Continuity of care

8. Prompt access to care

9. Comprehensiveness and care coordination

10. Template of the future

provide effective treatment for behavioral health conditions, support behavioral change interventions for patients and families, and connect to community partnerships to affect change at the community and population levels.

The models for primary care shared here begin with a team of people who integrate physical and behavioral health care to meet patients' needs. PCPs must embrace the shift to allow other team members to contribute in providing important tasks, such as health behavior change, panel management, and algorithm-based preventive care requirements. Primary care capacity can be increased by permitting licensed personnel to provide more aspects of care, by building standing order sets for paraprofessional staff, by teaching and encouraging patients in self-management techniques, and by implementing emerging technology to aid in the process (Bodenheimer and Smith 2013). This new care culture includes patients as team members in the design and then assures testing of new processes, explicit workflows, effective training, and expert patient coaching. Building shared goals, clear roles, mutual trust, and systems for effective communication as well as studying measurable processes and outcomes are the key principles of team-based health care defined by the Institute of Medicine Roundtable on Value & Science-Driven Health Care (Mitchell et al. 2012). Developing a culture that makes the patient and their family a part of the team, and the focus of the team, will help guide transformed collaborative care teams of the future to better health outcomes, better patient experience, and a better work environment.

THE PRIMARY CARE PROVIDER "CHAMPION" IN THE COLLABORATIVE CARE MODEL

One critical factor in the effectiveness of the Collaborative Care Model (CoCM) is the presence of a PCP "champion" on the team. This role includes possessing understanding and enthusiasm for the model, engaging patients into the treatment process, and then supporting both the patient and the BHP as they optimize the treatment plan (Whitebird et al. 2014). PCP champions must commit to the work, participate in the design and review of work processes, support implementation, educate physicians and other team members, and, most importantly, serve as a role model and cheerleader at various points when resistance occurs (Table 5–2). To practice outcome-changing and cost-effective collaborative care, there needs to be less of a focus on each staff member's traditional role and credentials and more attention paid to the functions that need to be performed and who can best provide these functions to address the patient as a whole. PCPs are very accustomed to being in charge of all aspects of care, and relinquishing control to allow new practices can be a challenge. The presence of a PCP champion can help to navigate these waters and help the team to provide more effective care.

PRIMARY CARE PROVIDER BUY-IN

One of the initial responses PCPs often state for reluctance in addressing patients' behavioral health conditions is their concern that this is a more time-consuming process—that it will slow them down and they will get behind in their schedule (Table 5–3). In reality, this is the situation in primary care practices already, and without the support of a team and a BHP, a 15-minute visit quickly becomes a 40- to 60-minute visit for the PCP alone, without any BHP support. Although the basic choreography of a patient's experience in the clinic or office is best when it is standardized, flexibility and a willingness to improve encounters with care team members is needed for optimal patient care and flow. For example, in a setting where truly collaborative care is the strategy, PCPs honor the tactical (cognitive and behavioral) strengths of all other team members. Because handling intense or complicated psychosocial issues is often time-consuming and disruptive to flow, in collaborative care, visits with the BHP often occur after the visit with the PCP (and frequently take at least as long as the visit with the PCP). However, when the care team or PCP is running behind, the patient (and team) may be best

TABLE 5–2. The primary care provider champion defined

Is committed to the goal of transforming the practice to the collaborative care model

May be in a formal or informal leadership role, demonstrates natural leadership skills, and has the respect of peer physicians and all team members

Understands behavioral health integration and a team-based care approach to primary care

Respects and demonstrates that all team roles are vitally important

Fosters trust among team members as they collaborate through appropriate sharing of the work to assure all indicated work is done for the patients

Is given time to truly lead the team and be the champion for the work— for example, attending meetings, helping to aid in implementation, educating physicians and other team members, helping to recruit the consulting psychiatrist

Source.   N. Jaekels Kamp, personal communication, August 14, 2015. From field notes collected in the research for Whitebird et al. (2014).

served if the BHP sees the patient first. Research has demonstrated PCP satisfaction with the CoCM (Levine et al. 2005); however, this new approach can be challenging for PCPs who may initially struggle with the requirement that they change the way they have traditionally provided care. In this way, the formal or informal leadership qualities of a PCP champion can be enormously valuable by helping to move their colleagues through these anticipated initial stages of resistance.

Some PCPs may express concerns regarding their liability when providing more behavioral health treatment than they are accustomed to or comfortable with, and they may use this as a reason not to participate in collaborative care. A reasonable response to this rationale is that PCPs who use collaborative care are doing gold standard treatment, with many more resources than they ever would have if trying to manage behavioral health conditions by themselves. Therefore, establishing a collaborative care team in a primary care clinic should actually reduce liability, not increase it, as long as all of the team members are performing in their roles as expected. Another role of the PCP champion will be to understand that this PCP concern may surface initially and to be prepared to explain the potential legal advantages to this model.

TABLE 5–3. Thoughts of a primary care provider before and after implementation of integrated care

Before implementation of integrated care	After experience with integrated care
This is going to slow me down.	This takes a load off my plate.
I don't have time to address one more problem.	This speeds me up.
I already do a good job of treating mental illness.	I always want to practice like this. I am giving better care to my patients.
This is going to drag on me like an anchor.	This gives me time to finish my notes.

ROLES OF THE PRIMARY CARE PROVIDER ON A COLLABORATIVE CARE TEAM

Leadership

The role of the PCP (including medical and osteopathic doctors, nurse practitioners, and physician assistants) on any effective collaborative care team includes multidimensional leadership closely linked to the patient and family as well as to the other team members. PCPs must commit to the ongoing emotional and psychological work of redefining their professional identity to encourage and celebrate meaningful participation of collaborative team members. In teams where this transition happens, PCPs can hand off work to skilled BHPs and other team members, including the patient, nursing staff, case management staff, medical assistants, and office staff in the primary care office. When the team aligns around shared goals and explicit, clear roles and workflows, the likelihood that patients receive all indicated care increases. Additionally, PCP champions who demonstrate steadiness in the presence of continuous innovation and near-constant change can dramatically impact the team's resilience. Pursuing relational coordination, including shared goals, shared knowledge, and mutual respect, matched with strategies of timeliness, accuracy, and a focus on problem solving will support high-functioning teams (Gittell et al. 2013).

Patient Engagement

Patients who understand the "why" of collaborative care are more likely to respond affirmatively to the "how": team-based care with a BHP and psychiatric consultant. Thus, the first task of the PCP is to highlight the links between body and mind, behavior and thoughts, and thoughts and emotions. Discussions about stress—externally and internally generated, eustress, and distress—lead naturally for many people to observations about coping, resilience, hardiness, and health. The PCP has an obligation to continually remind patients that humans have innate capacities for health, wellness, healing, and recovery—both in the body and the mind—and to invoke the desire shared by the PCP and patient to be and feel as well as possible, regardless of what is going on in the patient's mind, body, or life situation.

Harnessing the social power of the provider-patient relationship is probably the most effective means of engaging patients in this transformed care paradigm. The PCP's capacity to effectively redefine the nature of the caring relationship from "you and me" to "you and us" rests on the health of the relationship before the care team role changes occur. Many patients want to please a PCP that they trust and respect. The PCP who has taken the time to nurture a healing relationship that honors patients—as respected partners in care, experts of what change is wanted and needed in their lives, and those most knowledgeable of what has worked for them in the past—can leverage that trust to introduce and advocate for the participation of other team members, most notably the BHP.

The warm handoff from provider to the BHP is ideal, although there is some experimentation with electronic or "e-handoffs" to remote providers (see Chapter 1, "Elements of Effective Design and Implementation," and Chapter 4, "Behavioral Health Provider Essentials"). Having a PCP say, "I think it would help you to talk to someone on our care team that I have a lot of confidence in, and she's right down the hall—let's go see her," goes a long way toward persuading patients to agree to use behavioral health services (see Box 5–1 for additional scripts). Another approach is for the PCP and BHP to enter the room together at the beginning of the appointment and greet the patient. By entering the room together, introducing the concept of collaborative team-based care, and interacting effectively in support of each other's roles, patients get the sense of the comprehensiveness of the clinic's approach to their needs.

Box 5–1.   Examples of Provider-Patient Narratives for Warm Handoffs Between the PCP and BHP in the Exam Room

Example 1

PCP: This is our BHP, Margie, who I was telling you about.
BHP: Nice to meet you, Joe.

PCP: So, Joe has been struggling with pain and has not been able to do a lot of the things that he enjoys because of it, like playing with his grandchildren. He has been using more pain medication than I prescribed, so he tends to run out early. I worry about overuse of addictive and risky medication. I think that some of the treatments that you do so well will help him manage his pain better so that he doesn't run out of his medicine while still being able to do the things he enjoys.

BHP: Definitely, Joe. I have a little time right now if you can stay a bit longer. Would that be OK?

Example 2

PCP: Julie, this is my colleague, Margie, a member of our team who works with people on handling stress better.

BHP: Good to meet you, Julie.

PCP: Julie is now working two jobs and having a lot of headaches. She's taking up to 2,400 mg of ibuprofen daily, and I was telling her that I'm concerned about the safety of taking this much every day. Do you think she'd have fewer headaches if you shared some stress management techniques with her?

BHP: Well, it probably won't hurt, and I'd like to talk with her some about what else is going on in her life right now. Is that OK with you, Julie?

Source. Thanks to Margie Kaems, L.C.S.W., for Examples 1 and 2, personal communication, April 2016.

Example 3

Addressing chronic problems

"We have been working on this problem for a while. I have run the tests and I still need more information about what may be going on. Please excuse me while I go get our behavioral health team member to help us."

Addressing a problem that is mostly a behavioral health concern but the specific problem is unknown

"You deserve more support for _____ [*problem**] than I can give you right now, please excuse me; I'm going to get another team member to help us."

"Excuse me; you've started to tell me more about your situation, and I'm very concerned. You're telling me important information, but I'm going to interrupt our time to get another team member who can help me help you."

Addressing a specific behavioral health problem

"I can tell you've been depressed for a long time; I'm going to include our behavioral health provider in your care. I believe that [*in-*

sert patient's concern*] is part of the picture here and I'm going to include our BHP in your care."

*Examples of problems or concerns applicable to addressing a specific behavior: stress, exhaustion, loneliness, communication problems, worry, sadness, depression, managing pain, using substances, patient safety, frustration or anxiety, problems at school

Source. Thanks to Manuel Castro, M.D., for Example 3, personal communication, June 2016.

Prescribing Psychotropic Medications

Through the work of a high-functioning team that includes BHPs and consulting psychiatric providers, expert care of enduring benefit can be provided for a number of mild to moderate psychiatric disorders. Although many PCPs are comfortable prescribing medications for first- and sometimes second-line treatment of common disorders, such as depression and anxiety, there are significantly fewer who feel that they possess sufficient training to advance to more extensive augmentation and medication switching regimens, let alone prescribe treatment for severe or persistent mental illness. In particular, PCPs often avoid prescribing benzodiazepines, psychostimulants, or any antipsychotic medication on a chronic basis, regardless of the approval of the U.S. Food and Drug Administration. In the CoCM, PCPs apply evidence-based psychotropic medication interventions when indicated, with support from BHPs and psychiatric consultants who provide an opportunity for ongoing case-based learning with registry reviews of progress to track interventions.

An important task for the collaborative team is to provide real-time support for PCPs to extend their current level of knowledge and skill in psychotropic prescribing. Although often willing to initiate treatment, many PCPs frequently do not maximize treatment, leaving patients with partially treated or undertreated conditions and continued suffering along with a collateral impact on other health conditions (Wang et al. 2005). Partially treating or undertreating conditions can occur in several ways, including prescribing an insufficient dose of medication, terminating a treatment in less than the desirable time frame to elicit response (e.g., 4- to 6-week trials are often necessary for antidepressants), lacking knowledge of evidence-based prescribing algorithms for common disorders, and encountering difficulties in establishing a correct diagnosis. The CoCM provides a BHP on-site in the clinic and a psychiatric consultant available by phone and during the caseload review. This process can help the PCP confirm a diagnosis, decide what medication to start (or try next if a patient is already taking a medication that is not working), titrate a medication accurately, and augment or switch medications. The consultant can provide algorithms and psychotropic prescribing resources to help PCPs as they gain knowledge and grow more competent in prescribing (an example of a prescribing resource is available at https://aims.uw.edu/resource-library/commonly-prescribed-psychotropic-medications). Regularly scheduled brief educational sessions with the PCP can also be arranged and allow didactic as well as "stump the chump" question-and-answer opportunities. Programs such as Project ECHO (Extension for Community Healthcare Outcomes; http://echo.unm.edu) for psychiatric medication training can provide additional educational opportunities (see Chapter 1).

One of the most compelling reasons for the success of the CoCM is its measurement-based treatment-to-target approach. Using rating scales such as the Patient Health Questionnaire–9 (PHQ-9) to assess depression allows PCPs to measure response to treatment, which can alert them to the need to implement a change in strategy or continue with the current course of treatment, just as they do in monitoring diabetes or hypertension. The BHP keeps track of response to treatment in a registry, and during the weekly caseload review with the psychiatric consultant, additional recommendations for treatment adjustments can occur to continue the progression toward defined treatment targets. This method of measurement and treatment adjustment leads to improved outcomes, shorter duration of time to improvement, and better likelihood of reaching remission (Guo et al. 2015; see Figure 5–1).

Team Member and Collaborator

It is essential that PCPs function as team members. Collaborative care requires PCPs to serve in a role where they are not asked for specific directions for all interventions with the patient, as other team members have defined roles and the autonomy to step in and complete their specific tasks without the need for "permission" from the PCP to do so. Team members have duties defined by agreed-on evidence-based algorithms of care and are empowered to provide that care to the patient whenever appropriate. These actions may occur in the office before, during, or after a clinic visit, on the phone with the patient, or in other community settings. PCPs supporting team members as they work at the top of their license assures that all indicated care is given to the patient. The work of changing staff roles and workflows is challenging, and success hinges on shared knowledge, mutual respect, trust, and clear roles (Mitchell et al. 2012). Collaboration is required to meet the needs of the patients seeking care by planning and organizing approaches to reduce the chaos of a busy practice. As staff perform at the top of their license, PCPs must

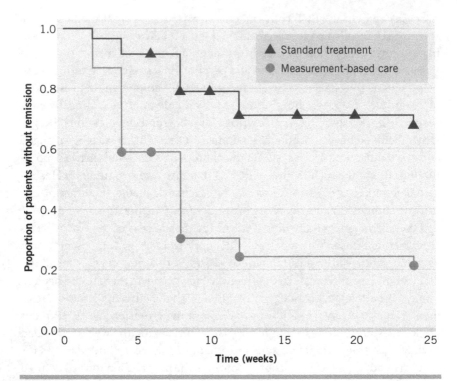

FIGURE 5–1.   Time to remission of symptoms using a measurement-based treatment-to-target approach.

Note.   The numbers of patients who achieved remission at 2, 4, 8, 12, and 24 weeks, respectively, were 2, 5, 12, 16, and 17 in the standard treatment group and 8, 25, 41, 44, and 45 in the measurement-based care group ($P < 0.001$).
Source.   Adapted from Guo T, Xiang YT, Xiao L, et al.: "Measurement-Based Care Versus Standard Care for Major Depression: A Randomized Controlled Trial With Blind Raters." *American Journal of Psychiatry* 172(10):1004–1013, 2015. Used with permission.

be supportive, take time to educate staff, and partner with team members to improve the processes when outcomes are less than expected. The MacColl Center for Health Care Innovation has built a team-based care resource Web site (www.improvingprimarycare.org) based on the lessons learned from studying over 300 exemplary primary health care sites in the United States and provides numerous tools and strategies for building high-functioning teams.

Working With BHPs

Close and trusting collaboration between the PCP and BHP is especially critical in the CoCM. The BHP has skills that can transfer some of the PCP's work to a team. Initially, a PCP may not fully trust the skills of the BHP and will be hesitant to turn over part of the delivery of patient care. Over time there can be a very meaningful transformation in the relationship, resulting in unique efficiencies that can contribute to better patient outcomes and improved PCP satisfaction with the workflow. A well-trained BHP offers effective evidence-based treatment strategies in the primary care setting, such as motivational interviewing, solution-focused brief therapy, and cognitive-behavioral therapy (see Chapter 4). Giving PCPs the opportunity to collaborate with BHPs in the care of emotionally fragile, hostile, or not-yet-engaged individuals provides a tremendous asset and time savings to the team, as well as allowing PCPs to learn new skills in managing difficult situations. BHPs often create additional relationships with the patient and family that can lead to opportunities for shared decision making and improved health. For patients with significant behavioral health issues, the BHP can serve as an indispensable link between the patient, the PCP, and the psychiatric consultant, allowing the PCP to move efficiently between patients while the BHP communicates with the psychiatric consultant. Without a team-based approach to delivering care, physical and behavioral health patient care gaps will be difficult to close efficiently. If not a village, improving patient health in primary care certainly takes an integrated team.

BHPs in the collaborative care setting address both behavioral health issues and nonbehavioral health problems by using multiple modalities. By offering effective behavioral change strategies to patients with tobacco use, obesity, sedentary lifestyle, pain management, and poor dental hygiene, BHPs help prevent the chronic diseases these behaviors engender. Using motivational interviewing skills, they guide patients and families through difficult decisions, such as end-of-life planning (http://theconversationproject.org). Interactive shared medical appointments covering prenatal care, effective parenting, and menopause and aging are also excellent venues to leverage the skills of a BHP in health promotion among those without significant behavioral health problems. By facilitating the process of setting achievable goals and overcoming barriers to reaching them, BHPs help patients develop the confidence and skill needed to cope with and address the daily challenges of living with chronic disease. Though this model of behavioral engagement is time-consuming, research has shown that it improves patient efficacy in managing chronic disease (Lorig et al. 1999). BHPs also provide resources for overcoming the many social determinants of health, but care must be taken in protecting BHPs' time to perform the tasks that require their level of licensure and allow other staff (such as community health workers and case managers) to assist as needed (see Chapter 4).

Working With Psychiatric Consultants

PCPs often spend less time with psychiatric consultants because of the ability of the BHP to serve as a conduit for the flow of information to and from the psychiatric consultant to the PCP. As mentioned in Chapter 6, "The Psychiatric Consultant," the most frequent requests for consultation by the PCP are for pharmacological interventions and diagnostic clarification (Norfleet et al. 2016). Similar to the BHP, the relationship and trust between the PCP and psychiatric consultant are crucial, and spending time together when possible is important to developing this relationship. The PCP decides whether to follow the psychiatric consultant's recommendations, orders all medications or additional labs or tests suggested, and remains in charge of the overall patient care. Knowing the psychiatric consultant is available as PCPs implement a treatment plan provides a sense of security—it allows PCPs to develop expertise and confidence to go beyond first-line treatments and successfully treat mild to moderate mental health and substance use disorders.

"There are two things in particular I like most about working with the psychiatrist. She always gives me a next step to try if the first recommendation does not work, which saves me time. The second thing is I feel like a better doctor because she has taught me something new."—K.R., pediatrician

---

POPULATION MANAGEMENT AND PLANNED CARE

Based on the groundbreaking work from the 1990s, exemplary primary care practices have learned to improve care by focusing on both the patients coming in to the clinic and those patients who are not actively seeking care (Wagner et al. 2001). High-functioning practices now assume accountability to improve health by partnering with the patient and family whether they are in the clinic, working, or in their home in the community. By studying the practice's population of patients, care teams identify the segments with prevalent and high-risk conditions and deliver evidence-based care. Using performance improvement tools such as registries and processes such as team huddles (see the section "Addressing Flow Before the Patient Arrives: Huddles" later in this chapter) to plan care, the health care team is informed and prepared to coordinate effective and collaborative care across the entire community's complex health care system and services (Wagner et al. 2006).

TABLE 5–4. Examples of high-risk population registries in integrated primary care practices

Diabetes	High-risk pregnancy
Hypertension	Attention-deficit/hyperactivity disorder
Depression	
Anxiety	Chronic pain
Asthma	Dyslipidemia
Cardiovascular disease	Substance use
Developmental delay	Anticoagulant patients
	Failure to thrive

What Is a Registry?

A *registry* is a current list of patients who meet one or more inclusion criteria and comprise a population of concern or focus (Table 5–4). Sometimes called "exception reports," by displaying only those patients who are currently due for an intervention, staff can focus on recommended interventions. A registry is an indispensable tool for tracking and managing care delivery for an entire group. In the era before electronic health records (EHRs), a registry might have been constructed by using a spreadsheet populated with data from manual chart audits. With an EHR, staff with report-writing savvy write code to process data farmed from discrete data fields in the EHR and create virtual or actual reports relatively quickly for use at the time of care (for more on registries, see Chapters 1, 4, and 6).

How to Use Registry Information

Outreach

Outreach is the antidote to the "lost to follow-up" status. A current registry is key to identifying clients in the population of focus whose outcomes are missing the mark or who are overdue for care. From an operational or practice management perspective, a registry is indispensable for proactively managing an appointment schedule with vacancies by scheduling patients who need specified interventions. With some EHRs, a skilled information technology team can create a sophisticated outreach tool that identifies all patients belonging to one or more populations of focus who are overdue or coming due for a service (visit, screening, or study) based on evidence-based algorithms for care. The responsibility for running the tool and working it typically falls to office technicians who document their efforts in the tool and, automatically, in the EHR.

In-Reach

In-reach is a means for offering all care deemed necessary to reach the goals that really matter for patients being seen that day. An effective version of an in-reach tool provides the information needed by the care team to guide decisions around which clinical issues they want to focus on during a visit. Although the actual focus of the clinical encounter is decided with the patient, the in-reach tool is indispensable for planning care. These "care planners" are linked to the outreach registries, so the work of the office staff is matched to the work of clinicians seeing the patient when they arrive for a visit. During a 10-minute huddle before the first patient visit of the day, the PCP and the medical assistant quickly review the registry, identifying what additional preparation (e.g., repeat measurement tools such as the PHQ-9, lab or consultation results) may be needed before the patient care encounter. Usually an even briefer huddle occurs separately with the BHP who has identified which patients, of all the patients being seen by the care team, they most want to meet (see Chapter 4). The end of the care session is typically the best time for the care team to "debrief" and discuss what needs to be done before the patient's next visit.

COLLABORATIVE CARE WORKFLOWS IN PRIMARY CARE

Efficient workflow (hereafter, "flow") makes the wheels of primary care turn smoothly and is an important consideration when implementing collaborative care. Members of the care team own discrete tasks, and each is not only responsible for the consistent and prompt completion of these tasks but also for the handoffs among team members. Obviously, physical co-location of all team members makes for more efficient flow. When the physical layout of the office or clinic precludes co-location, some other means of facilitating interaction is needed (e.g., a pager, mobile phone, walkie-talkie, or whiteboard at each team member's desk). Optimal flow occurs when appointments are scheduled (i.e., walk-in visits are discouraged), the care team stays on time, and at least one member of the team is explicitly responsible for managing flow. A proactive medical assistant or nurse with solid management skills is well suited for this role.

Workflow Considerations

Addressing Flow Before the Patient Arrives: Huddles

Ideally, the care team, including the PCP, meets (huddles) before the start of a care session, anticipating outstanding or imminent care needs and recommended preventive or screening services (see also discussions of huddles in Chapter 3, "Team Development and Culture," and Chapter 4, "Behavioral Health Provider Essentials"). Screening is the process by which significant problems are uncovered before signs and symptoms occur, and the huddle can be used as a reminder to have appropriate screenings completed. These care team tasks must be integrated into the visit when the patient arrives with his or her agenda. In many settings, PCPs outnumber BHPs, so the huddle is a good time for the BHP to identify which patient(s) they need to see that day.

Addressing Flow When the Patient Arrives

Just as every clinical encounter has a flow, each has a purpose (often multiple). Ultimately, the care team's primary responsibility is to provide the care the patient wants and needs at the time he or she wants and needs it. Sometimes satisfactorily addressing the patient's stated reason for the encounter achieves this goal. At other times, especially when there are undiscovered or unaddressed social, behavioral, or psychological comorbidities, this response is insufficient.

In a visit initiated by the patient (or family), the patient's agenda should "drive" the encounter. Nonetheless, the care team integrates its own concerns, informing the conversation around the goal(s) for the visit. The PCP is responsible for framing at the outset patient complaints and concerns within the paradigm of the biopsychosocial (body-mind-community) model of health. Done well, this discussion increases the patient's receptivity to meeting and working with the BHP and other members of the team (e.g., a case manager knowledgeable about community resources). Handoffs between members of the care team are best when they are explicit ("I'm going to ask my medical assistant to come in now and draw your blood") and warm (both members present with the patient simultaneously); see the following case example.

Case Example: Addressing Flow—Prioritizing Issues During an Integrated Visit

A patient scheduled for a routine diabetes checkup comes into the primary care exam room reporting left hip pain. The PCP also notes the patient's annual PHQ-9 screening score is high, at a score of 18. How does the PCP fit the PHQ-9 review, depression discussion, and a new complaint of hip pain into an appointment originally for a diabetes follow-up?

A beauty and strength of primary care is comprehensiveness in the context of continuity (the relationship is expected to be longitudinal, ideally over the span of the patient's life). In abiding by the principle of relationship-centered care, the PCP is obligated to address the patient's acute complaint (pain) while simultaneously addressing the concern that could be impacting both the pain and diabetes—the likely presence of a mood disorder. Here's how the conversation might go after the PCP gathers additional information about the pain and assures the patient that her complaint will be thoroughly evaluated and treated.

PCP: I can see that your hip is really bothering you.

Patient: Oh doc, I can barely walk. I couldn't sleep at all last night because of the pain.

PCP: That sounds bad enough that I would like to talk to you a bit more about it, do an examination, and come up with a plan. Is that OK with you?

Patient: Yes, please. I can't live like this.

PCP: I am confident we can help you feel better. I have another concern that is just as important to me. It's about that form you filled out. Is it OK if we talk about that right now?

Patient: Just as long as you take care of the pain.

PCP: For sure. This form is a tool we use to identify patients who might be suffering from depression. Your score is pretty high, and I'm concerned you may have depression.

Patient: You'd feel down too if you had this pain. It's bad enough I have to check my blood sugar and can't eat the foods I like (starts to cry).

PCP (*grabs a tissue and offers it to the patient*): I promise we'll deal with your hip pain today. Depression makes everything worse, including pain. I have a colleague I trust who's helped many of my patients who are struggling with pain and sadness. Would it be OK if I asked her to help us?

Patient: Yeah, I guess if you think it would help.

PCP: Let me see if she's available and I'll be right back, OK? When the two of you are finished talking, she'll call me back in and we can talk some more about your hip pain and do an examination. By the way, I looked at the blood test you completed before this visit and your diabetes is OK for now. Let's focus on these other problems.

Patient: Whatever you say. You're the doctor.

Documentation and Information Sharing

The documentation requirements around the nature and content of the work done by BHPs often require the creation of a separate note, even when the care is collaborative. It is vital that the BHP's notes are not "hidden" from the view of the PCPs so they can see the behavioral interventions that are occurring, including any discussions with the psychiatric consultant, and can support and encourage behavioral change and adherence to treatment. The BHP is often the conduit of information to and from the psychiatric consultant and PCP, and it is important that the information from this exchange be included in the BHP's documentation or communicated to the PCP through a workflow "tasking" function in the EHR.

ADULT VISITS IN COLLABORATIVE CARE

Visits in adult primary care may be characterized by the nature of the concern or condition needing attention (e.g., acute care, chronic care, well and/ or preventive care, administrative follow-up), the qualifications of the person providing the care (e.g., medical assistant, nurse, or PCP), or the manner in which the care is delivered (e.g., telephonically, face-to-face individual, face-to-face group). In most primary care settings in the United States, the majority of encounters with nonelderly adults are face-to-face visits, with individuals unaccompanied by a family member or other support person.

Detection of Mental Health and Substance Use Disorders Through Routine Screening

Screening may occur with any visit type. In the absence of literacy concerns, valid patient self-report measures are more time efficient than those requiring an interview by a clinician. The process may start at the front desk with the receptionist documenting that the screening tool was given, followed by the medical assistant making sure that the completed screening tool arrives with patients when they enter the exam room. The medical assistant scores the instrument, decides whether another back-office tool is needed (e.g., PHQ-9 in the case of a positive PHQ-2), and alerts the PCP or BHP regarding the abnormal screening result (see additional screening tools in Chapter 1).

Symptom-Driven Diagnosis of a New Disorder

A second means of discovery occurs when the PCP may suspect a behavioral health disorder during the course of a visit. A screening tool targeting the suspected condition is an efficient means of both diagnosing it and quantifying its severity. In primary care, nonbipolar depression is a good example. The PCP may be able to leave the room to recruit the help of the BHP while the patient completes the PHQ-9.

Case Example

MG is an overweight 34-year-old Latina with chronic low back pain, a poorly defined seizure disorder, and carpal tunnel syndrome. She works at a fast-food restaurant full-time. When she's home, she cares for her blind, diabetic father and her three children. She presents to the clinic, 15 minutes late, with intermittent chest pain and with left arm numbness that started 2 weeks earlier. Noting that the patient is due for an annual substance use and depression screen, the receptionist gives the patient a six-question screen to complete while she is waiting to be taken back by the medical assistant. The medical assistant, noting the chief complaint, speaks with the nurse about the patient's chest pain, who interrupts the PCP to see if he wants an electrocardiogram (ECG) done. While the nurse takes additional history, the medical assistant obtains the ECG and then takes it to the PCP, who tells her that it is normal. When the medical assistant returns to the room to remove the ECG leads, she notes that the substance use screen is negative, but the PHQ-2 is positive. She asks the patient to complete the PHQ-9 while she awaits her PCP, who is now 25 minutes behind schedule.

The nurse enters the exam room and scores the PHQ-9, notes that it is high (23 out of 27 possible points), and alerts the BHP. The BHP checks in with the patient and discovers that MG's youngest daughter will soon be hospitalized for surgery. MG cannot vocalize a particular concern or worry, but cries as she speaks of the upcoming surgery. When asked about self-care practices that help her cope with stressful situations, she mentions that she has not had more than a day off each week from work in more than a year. The BHP explores with the patient what she thinks might help, and the patient decides that she will ask her boss for a week off around the time of her daughter's surgery. MG also decides to increase the frequency of Zumba, an activity she sometimes does with coworkers at the end of their shifts.

Before the PCP enters the room, the BHP checks in with him regarding the situation and plan. The PCP briefly interviews and examines the patient, discusses possible reasons for the chest pain and arm symptoms, tells her that he suspects she is having panic attacks, affirms the wisdom of the plan jointly created by the patient and the BHP, and decides to check some blood work. He then offers the patient a prescription to calm anxiety. MG declines, stating that she is feeling better and does not want to mix that medicine with the medicine she takes for pain. On subsequent visits she retakes the PHQ-9, which has decreased to a score of 12 by her next visit 1 month later. The BHP continues to track her progress in the registry, and treatment adjustments are made as needed.

Follow-Up of an Established Behavioral Health Disorder Managed in the Primary Care Setting

Follow-up can be arranged proactively by use of a registry (see the section "What Is a Registry" earlier in this chapter), with the receptionist contacting the patient to schedule an appointment, or extemporaneously during a huddle (provided the disorder is being tracked and identified during the previsit huddle). The PCP and BHP together decide on an approach for checking in with the patient, with the understanding the plan may change if a crisis arises that prevents either from seeing the patient. The huddle is a good time for the BHP or PCP to enlist the help of another team member (e.g., medical assistant or case manager) in gathering information (e.g., a PHQ-9 or urine drug screening test) before the patient is seen by a clinician.

Follow-Up of an Established Behavioral Health Disorder Managed in a Specialty Mental Health Care Setting

The BHP is often best suited for acting as a liaison and care coordinator or manager for patients who are jointly followed in both the primary care and specialty mental health care settings. Creating a coherent care plan with goals shared by as many as four persons—the patient, therapist, psychiatric prescriber, and PCP—poses significant but manageable challenges.

PEDIATRIC VISITS IN COLLABORATIVE CARE

Many behavioral health conditions in children are now being managed by PCPs in integrated settings, presenting an opportunity for collaborative care. A recent meta-analysis of existing randomized controlled clinical trials in pediatric patients indicated that integrating care for mental health problems in primary care for children and adolescents leads to significant improvement in child and adolescent behavioral health outcomes. The effects were stronger in treatment trials than prevention trials, and the strongest effects were seen in collaborative care interventions with evidence-based medication algorithms and evidence-based psychotherapy (Asarnow et al. 2015).

Types of Pediatric Visits

Ideally, in the initial visit the PCP and BHP jointly meet the patient and family and introduce them to the integrated model and care team, including the role of the BHP. Screening for particular behavioral health concerns occurs, and treatment is implemented as indicated. Education is provided, and the team, which includes the patient and family, develop next steps as partners in the treatment process. At follow-up visits, there is review of ongoing behavioral health concerns, response and adherence to the treatment plan, and reevaluation of the care plan. Much like the adult patient workflow described earlier in this chapter, proactive planning for the daily schedule of patients should include a huddle to review specific care needs for patients and required action to prepare for the visit (including repeat measurement of behavioral health conditions with valid tools) based on information garnered during this process. Table 5–5 presents a list of the types of pediatric visits where collaboration could occur.

Bright Futures is a national health promotion and prevention initiative, led by the American Academy of Pediatrics and supported by the Maternal Child and Health Bureau, Health Resources and Services Administration (https://brightfutures.aap.org/Pages/default.aspx). It provides theory-based and evidence-driven guidance for all preventive care screenings and well-

---

TABLE 5–5. Standard pediatric visits that present an opportunity for an integrated visit

---

1. Well-child and adolescent visits

2. Sports physicals

3. Chronic care visits: asthma, seizures, diabetes, obesity, special needs

4. Acute sick visits

5. Behavioral health conditions: depression, anxiety, attention-deficit/ hyperactivity disorder

6. Immunizations

7. Weight checks

8. Family planning and reproductive health visits for adolescents

---

child visits that most pediatricians implement in their well-child visits. During well-child visits, health maintenance concerns such as diet and nutrition, sleep, growth and development, hearing and vision screening, and immunizations are addressed. A comprehensive history, including diet and nutrition and sleep, is performed as well as measurements including vital signs, sensory screening for vision and hearing, and developmental and behavioral screening. A comprehensive physical exam including an oral health exam and procedures such as newborn screening, hemoglobin, lead and tuberculosis screening, and other laboratory screening procedures are performed if clinically indicated. Anticipatory guidance for parents regarding these health promotion and injury and disease prevention strategies can be provided by both the PCP and the BHP. Some examples of anticipatory guidance include healthy food choices and exercise, use of helmets and other safety equipment, sun and water safety, handwashing, disease prevention, sleep hygiene, toilet training, and age-appropriate discipline. Well-child visits are ideal for integrated encounters as developmental and behavioral screenings occur, and BHPs can help address normal development concerns, such as sleep, discipline, and other parenting concerns, in addition to distinct psychiatric disorders. Because there are several screening tools to be administered, and often children will be receiving immunizations at the end of their visits, it is imperative that the entire care team works efficiently and with knowledge of and regard for the other member's roles and responsibilities in order for the patient to receive all necessary services.

Other appointments include sports physicals, which present an opportunity for screening for depression or substance use. Children with chronic medical conditions often have coexisting behavioral health concerns either directly or indirectly related to their medical conditions, which makes this encounter ideal for integrated visits. During acute sick visits to the PCP, children are often not feeling well and can be scared or anxious, especially when a procedure needs to performed. This holds true for immunization visits as well. The BHP can be a welcomed resource for the child and parents, helping ease the child's anxiety and thereby facilitating the performance of necessary procedures and interventions. Finally, reproductive health visits are another ideal integrated encounter, during which the BHP can help the adolescent with issues such as making good choices about sexuality and compliance with contraceptive methods and disease prevention.

Psychopharmacology

With the scarcity of child psychiatrists in many suburban and rural areas, more and more often pediatricians are being called on to manage behavioral health conditions such as attention-deficit/hyperactivity disorder (ADHD), depression, and anxiety disorders. In addition, fewer than 40% of children and adolescents with a behavioral health diagnosis will seek specialty care outside of their PCP (Wang et al. 2005). Many pediatricians feel undertrained to treat these conditions, but with a supportive collaborative care team including a BHP and a psychiatric consultant as well as resources for diagnosis, management, and psychopharmacology (see Seattle Children's *Primary Care Principles for Child Mental Health*, www.seattlechildrens.org/pdf/PAL/WA/WA-care-guide.pdf), many of these conditions can be successfully managed with increasing confidence by PCPs.

Pediatric Workflow

With very tight schedules, PCPs need efficient workflows in order to provide high-quality services to their patients. Many measurements and screenings are required at each type of pediatric visit, and PCPs often are rushed to complete the encounter. Some factors that could help facilitate a high-quality encounter in each of these scenarios include screening tools and measurements completed before patients enter the exam room (Table 5–6). Measurements and screenings can be discussed at the morning huddle so support staff are aware of their role in administering these tools and in caring for the patient's needs. Patients should be instructed to come early in order to complete the necessary screening tools before their encounter.

Case Example

A 13-year-old white male presented for a new patient visit for behavioral health services because of a referral from restorative justice after community

TABLE 5–6. Population-based pediatric screening tools

Age	Tool
2–60 months	Ages and Stages Questionnaire, Third Edition (ASQ-3; Schonhaut et al. 2013; http://agesandstages.com)
16–30 months	Modified Checklist for Autism in Toddlers (M-CHAT; Robins et al. 2014)
61 months to 11 years	Strengths and Difficulties Questionnaire (SDQ; Goodman 1997)
6–12 years	Vanderbilt ADHD Diagnostic Rating Scale (parent and teacher versions; Wolraich et al. 2003)
12–17 years	Patient Health Questionnaire for Adolescents (PHQ-A; Johnson et al. 2002) CRAFFT—substance use (stands for Car, Relax, Alone, Forget, Friends, Trouble questions; Knight et al. 2002)

Note.   ADHD = attention-deficit/hyperactivity disorder.

vandalism. He had a historical diagnosis of ADHD. He was taking guanfacine 1.5 mg bid, which was prescribed by a previous PCP. His ADHD symptoms were not well controlled, evidenced by his Vanderbilt Assessment Scales score, and he was experiencing medication side effects, such as fatigue, daytime somnolence, dizziness, and palpitations. He was noted to have bradycardia with a heart rate of 56. An ECG was ordered, which again showed significant bradycardia. With the help of the BHP and the psychiatric consultant, he was weaned off of the guanfacine, and extended-release methylphenidate was added. He tolerated this medication much better with no further side effects and better control of his ADHD symptoms.

Other processes can facilitate a more even flow and can be considered based on available space and resources. These include the following:

1. The team enters the room together whenever possible to introduce the concept of collaborative care as a high-quality, evidence-based approach to care. This limits confusion and multiple questions about care team member's roles.
2. One of the care team members takes the lead in the visit to streamline the encounter process. This can be done by either the PCP or the BHP.

3. Each PCP/BHP team has the time and proper training to work with each other and develop a flow or "dance," as each partner engages and participates in the encounter. For example, BHPs can help engage patients' siblings during a focused history by the PCP, allowing the PCP and parent the time to review necessary history. In addition, the BHP may review behavioral health screening tools with a parent while the PCP is examining the child. This approach allows for maximum efficiency because each member of the team is addressing multiple issues and there is little downtime during the encounter.

4. If an acute behavioral health issue is identified and needs to be addressed, the BHP can provide brief intervention with the patient and family at the end of the encounter, allowing the PCP to step out of the room and move on to other patients.

PRIMARY CARE PROVIDERS IN BEHAVIORAL HEALTH SETTINGS

For the past decade, a strong case has been made for placing primary care within a behavioral health setting (Mauer 2006), such as a community mental health center (CMHC), creating a medical home for patients with serious mental illness (SMI). These patients have a lifespan shortened by 20 to 30 years (Colton and Manderscheid 2006) and are dying of preventable diseases, such as cardiovascular disease, infectious diseases, and tobacco-related disorders, as well as having cancer detected in later stages (de Hert et al. 2011). Dubbed "reverse integration" or "bidirectional integration," this approach ascribes to the Francis Bacon principle "If the mountain won't come to Muhammad, then Muhammad must go to the mountain." (See Table 2 in the appendix, "Performance and Outcome Measures for Integrated Care," for several examples of outcome measures for the integrated physical care of patients with SMI.)

In general, persons with SMI engage much better with CMHCs; however, these clinics have not been able to deliver the high-quality primary care that this population requires. Entities that are bringing primary care into CMHCs are showing a great deal of promise in caring for the most difficult to treat patients (Kern 2015). However, there are some unique challenges associated with this approach (Scharf et al. 2013).

Engagement

Persons with SMI have a much lower rate of engagement with high-quality primary care, despite the fact that they carry a much higher disease burden (McCabe and Leas 2008). Also, because of their high level of medical, mental

TABLE 5–7. Patient and provider factors that may inhibit engagement in patients with serious mental illness

Patient factors	Provider factors
Lack of motivation; apathy	Lack of knowledge or experience with specific disorders
Cognitive impairment (poor judgment)	
	Attributing physical symptoms to mental illness and therefore missing the diagnosis
Lack of perceived need for health care	
Comorbidity (substance abuse)	High no-show rates, lack of follow-up, longer length of visit
Poor social and communication skills	
	Fear of symptomatic patients
Fear and distrust of the medical system	

health, substance abuse, and socioeconomic complications, these persons have an even greater need for an integrated team-based approach. The low rate of engagement with primary care is multifactorial (Table 5–7). Traditionally, primary care offices have been volume and payer driven, reflecting the needs of their financial bottom line. Persons with SMI typically have poorer insurance coverage and a much greater degree of medical complexity. Simply put, there is not a very good "bang for your buck" with this patient population for a traditional PCP office. Many PCPs are reluctant to engage with the SMI population because of the perception that these patients do not have a "physical illness," or PCPs may write off complaints as "not real," a facet of the patient's mental illness (Lester et al. 2005).

Physical Space

Primary care has a much larger footprint than behavioral health. Typically, PCPs work in multiple rooms (three rooms per provider for maximal efficiency), whereas behavioral health providers only need one room. Plumbing for exam rooms, laboratory facilities, and the location of medical supplies are just a few differences in the layouts of their respective workplaces (Table 5–8). Examination rooms for patients with SMI ideally should be larger than in a traditional PCP office to accommodate the number of persons involved in their care and to avoid intrusion into the personal space of the patient. Having several chairs in the exam room helps to make personnel that accompany the patient more comfortable and facilitates warm handoffs. For

---

TABLE 5–8. Equipping the exam room (items stored in a secure location)

Sphygmomanometer: with small, medium, large, and extra-large cuff

Scale

Otoscope and ophthalmoscope

Stethoscope

Reflex hammer

Nail clippers

No. 10, 11, and 15 scalpels

Tongue depressors, gauze pads, hand sanitizer, alcohol wipes, nonlatex gloves

Access to electronic health record, laptop, and other electronic aids

---

many patients with SMI, having an examination room that is warm and friendly helps them to relax and feel more comfortable. The room should be large enough to not feel crowded, have good lighting, and ideally have a sink for hand washing.

Many patients with SMI have histories of negative experiences in the sterile environments of hospitals. Having art or pictures on the walls produced by peer wellness coaches, or signs that remind the patient to focus on simple goals, such as "Eat five servings per day of vegetables or fruit," "Try to walk for 30 minutes each day," and "Try to quit smoking," are well received by patients. Anatomical depictions of various disease states should be avoided because they can frighten patients already plagued by delusions and hallucinations and bizarre ways of interpreting the world around them.

Working With Psychiatric Providers in a Mental Health Setting

For PCPs working in a mental health setting, interacting with psychiatric providers can be a very mutually rewarding experience. A reciprocal back-and-forth develops as each clinician is able to appreciate the other's perspective regarding the care of the patient. In evaluating patients with SMI in hospitals and typical clinic environments, the physical health provider may assume that symptoms are a manifestation of mental illness, whereas the mental health provider fears that the symptoms are a manifestation of a physical illness. In the integrated environment, however, there is an opportunity to look together at the patient as a whole and for each clinician to explain his or her understanding and idea. A typical example is a patient with bipolar disorder, well controlled on olanzapine, who presents with meta-bolic syndrome in a primary care visit. The PCP may want to tell the patient that the olanzapine is a "bad medication that is causing your diabetes." How-ever, through close coordination with the psychiatric providers, the clinician can determine if other medications have been tried and failed or if the olan-zapine is the only medication found to be effective in this patient and more intensive treatment of the diabetes is necessary.

Physical Exam

With the exception of pediatric patients, PCPs take for granted that patients will allow a physical examination and cooperate with procedures. In the be-havioral health world, however, physically touching the patient is tradition-ally seen as a taboo. For patients with a history of sexual trauma or physical abuse and SMI, even something as benign as taking vital signs becomes something to negotiate. It is not uncommon for the very first physical health visit to be a home visit or for the patient to come into the office just to see the exam room. It may not be until the third or fourth visit that the patient allows a stethoscope to be used and then insists it be placed on the outside of his or her shirt. The following case provides an example of an encounter with a patient with a severe mental illness.

Case Example: A PCP's Approach to the Physical Exam in a Reluctant Patient

A 57-year-old woman with schizophrenia presented to the CMHC primary care clinic. Staff at the group home had reported worsening body odor. She had not removed her socks in weeks. She asked all the staff to leave the ex-amination room and indicated that only I could do the exam. She had five layers of old socks to be removed, layers of dirt, dead skin, tinea pedis, and toenails that were 4 inches long and encrusted with dirt. It took 45 minutes to soak and clean her feet and remove the nails with a trimmer. She would only allow me to use water and hydrogen peroxide, no betadine or alcohol. We offered her three pairs of fresh black tube socks (she only dresses in black), and she allowed us to take the old socks in exchange.

Team-Based Care in the Behavioral Health Setting

As discussed earlier in this section, team-based care is crucial to caring for the SMI population. Fortunately, CMHCs have also been working with teams for many years and are very facile when privacy barriers are removed and pri-mary care is placed on their team. For the PCP, the challenge of overwhelming patient complexity can be offset by team-based care and the realization that you can delegate to other members of the team by warm handoffs. For example, it is not uncommon for a PCP to see a patient with poorly controlled SMI and also having untreated, undiagnosed chronic medical problems, such as diabetes, chronic obstructive pulmonary disease, hyperlipidemia, and hypertension along with a substance use disorder, lack of housing, and lack of health care insurance standing in the way of effective treatment. Having a cohesive team that consists of care managers, psychiatrists, tobacco cessation specialists, diabetic nurse educators, substance use counselors, and service coordinators allows the PCP to get at the root of social and behavioral health problems that make treatment of the underlying medical condition possible. For example, a patient may have a blood pressure of 160/100 (high) and a hemoglobin A_{1c} at 9.5 (high), have no housing, and be actively drinking alcohol and exhibiting psychotic symptoms. Enlisting the team to stabilize housing and mental illness first allows the possibility that the patient can then shift focus to be able to receive advice on diet and medications once these social issues are remedied. It may be difficult for a traditional PCP to delay these treatment steps, but the reality of this population is that the psychosocial issues often must be addressed first in order to make any useful steps toward health behavior change.

The "Right Stuff"

Caring for the complex medical, behavioral health, and social needs of a population with SMI takes a team effort. So who are the "right people" for this work? A typical team for an integrated practice within a CMHC would best consist of a PCP, a psychiatric provider, a care manager, a peer wellness coach, a medical assistant, and a medical secretary.

The PCP most suited for this setting would be one who has a great deal of experience working with the patient population, as well as a generally flexible attitude. Often these clinicians have worked in underserved settings such as the Indian Health Service or Federally Qualified Health Centers. In those environments, they may have discovered an interest in helping those with mental illness and substance abuse problems. A willingness to learn new approaches to caring for patients with SMI is required, as well as a mindset of "harm reduction" instead of comprehensive management for the patient population.

Many psychiatric providers welcome an opportunity to collaborate with PCPs. An open style of communication and mindset toward a team effort is essential. Neither provider should hesitate to call the other with questions and discuss cases with each other. Struggling over each other's clinical territory can occur and is counterproductive. It is important for psychiatric providers to embrace new learning, including having the PCP help to expand their comfort in prescribing and managing medications (like metformin for diabetes or prediabetes) for common medical conditions.

Case Example: A Collaboration Between PCP and Psychiatrist

A patient with schizophrenia presents to a PCP's office, stable for the past year on olanzapine after failing multiple other medications, and the patient is found to have new-onset diabetes. The PCP notes a 40-pound weight increase in the past year and does the appropriate blood work, nutritional counseling, and initiation of treatment. The PCP might suggest to the patient that he would like to discuss with the patient's psychiatric provider the possibility of changing the olanzapine to another medication. In a trusting PCP–psychiatric provider relationship, the PCP can relate information to the psychiatrist in an informative way that asks if alternatives to olanzapine might exist for the patient and, if not, perhaps a dosage reduction or addition of a medication to offset the iatrogenic effects (in this case olanzapine) of the efficacious medication. The psychiatrist sees this as new information that may benefit the patient and not a threat to the clinical choice of medication. It is also a learning opportunity for both parties.

The care manager is a new addition to the CMHC team, filling a different role than traditional psychiatric nurses. The role requires someone with the heart of a teacher and the resourcefulness of a social worker, as well as medical skills and the ability to multitask. Care managers should also be flexible and comfortable working in a faster-paced environment. Typically, one care manager will assist multiple providers, delivering education on diabetes in one room, tobacco cessation in another, and advance directives in yet another. Care managers can have a background as a therapist, social worker, or nurse and are best used when they are doing direct care, which is typically in the office but sometimes can be in the community. They also manage the registry, keeping track of who needs what intervention next and who is not engaging or following through with care.

Psychopharmacology

For the PCP who works within a CMHC, it is essential to become familiar and comfortable with psychopharmacology and the metabolic side effects associated with many of these medications. This includes knowledge of medication-assisted treatment for a variety of substance use disorders, such as opiate and alcohol addiction. A list of medications that are commonly used today in CMHCs and serve as a good resource for the PCP is available at: https://aims.uw.edu/resource-library/commonly-prescribed-psychotropic-medications.

COLLABORATIVE CARE WITH PATIENTS OF DIFFERENT CULTURES

It has been well established that racial and ethnic minority groups in the United States have less access to health care and mental health services (Wang et al. 2005). In addition, minority groups are more likely to receive lower-quality care (Alegría et al. 2008), are more likely to have higher inpatient hospitalization and emergency department utilization, and less likely to use community mental health services (Samnaliev et al. 2009). Decreased access and utilization of care among ethnic minorities are attributed to delayed treatment seeking (Wang et al. 2005) and premature termination of treatment (Fortuna et al. 2010). In addition, there tends to be a preference for nontraditional mental health services (Abe-Kim et al. 2007). These factors influence how and why ethnic, underserved minority groups receive care and argue against an actual lower prevalence of disorders (Lee et al. 2011). Despite some evidence of lower prevalence rates of mood and anxiety disorders among many racial and ethnic minorities compared with whites (Kessler et al. 2005), other research suggests that these illnesses and disorders are often more severe, persistent, and disabling (Breslau et al. 2005). Thus, decreased access to timely, coordinated, continuous, and comprehensive health care tailored to the needs of racial and ethnic minority communities leads to a significant burden of disease, frustration exacerbated by the fragmentation of the health care, and ultimately greater health care costs.

In many cultures, the stigma of having a behavioral health condition is great, and receiving treatment in the privacy of the primary care setting is a welcome alternative to outside referral. Collaborative care has the potential to reduce racial and ethnic disparities with respect to mental and physical health by improving access, quality of care, and clinical outcomes (Davis et al. 2011; van Steenbergen-Weijenburg et al. 2010; Woltmann et al. 2012). Culturally adapted interventions using BHPs can improve treatment initiation, patient activation, and self-management among minorities with limited English proficiency and limited health literacy.

Latinos

In San Diego, integrated care models were successfully used in low-income predominantly Spanish-speaking Latino populations, combining Improving Mood—Promoting Access to Collaborative Treatment (IMPACT) depression care management with an existing diabetes care management program. This research demonstrated that this kind of combined approach is both effective and cost-effective with this population (Gilmer et al. 2008).

Asian Americans

Research shows that the CoCM improves the response to depression treatment for Asian Americans. Patients treated in the clinic that provided more culturally sensitive treatment received less psychotropic medications (Ratzliff et al. 2013).

African Americans

Collaborative care models have shown promise for addressing depression and other common mental health disorders in ethnic minorities including African Americans (Cooper et al. 2013; Unützer et al. 2002). Studies show improved outcomes and quality of mental health services (Interian et al. 2010; Miranda et al. 2003). The collaborative care models show the potential for reducing racial/ethnic disparities in mental health service access and utilization, quality of care, and clinical outcomes (Davis et al. 2011; Interian et al. 2010; Miranda et al. 2003; van Steenbergen-Weijenburg et al. 2010; Woltmann et al. 2012). More research is needed to understand efficacy in individual minority populations (Collins 2012).

American Indians

Although there is no current research on the efficacy of CoCM in American Indian (including Alaskan) populations, holistic, integrated care models have been identified as one way to address the challenges of delivering effective health care to American Indian populations (Napoli 2002). In 2006 the Indian Health Service developed a partnership with the Institute for Healthcare Improvement to implement one of the first collaborative care models to improve patient care throughout American Indian communities served by the Indian Health Service. Uncomplicated depression was one of the conditions included, and the pilot sites saw improvements in health outcomes and patient-provider relationships.

Case Example: Introducing Integrated Care to an American Indian Patient

A 34-year-old American Indian presented to the clinic with concerns about not sleeping, feeling on edge frequently, and having "visions" since being discharged from the military. He described his visions to the PCP as vivid and unsettling, usually of the people and experiences he had in the Middle East. He tried working excessively to preoccupy himself, but he was recently fired from his job for being late. He admitted to self-medicating with alcohol frequently to deal with the visions. The PCP expressed concern with what the patient was telling her and told him that she had seen this fairly frequently with other American Indian veterans. The PCP told him that she was concerned and wanted to help him, then asked if she could bring in a colleague to help. He replied, "No, I don't want to tell anyone anything else. I don't think they will understand." She mentioned that her colleague had helped several other people with similar situations and that she would stay in the room. If he felt uncomfortable at any point, she could ask the colleague to leave. He agreed, and she went across the hall to get the BHP. The interview proceeded, and the patient was set up with monthly integrated follow-ups with the BHP and the PCP. A brief consultation was also made to the psychiatric consultant to confirm the diagnosis of posttraumatic stress disorder. After the first follow-up visit, the BHP coordinated a 60-day and inpatient rehab stint at a facility that was focused on providing services to American Indian patients.

CONCLUSION

Anticipating the inevitable health care change described at the start of this chapter, robust team-based care—which includes a PCP, a BHP, and a psychiatric consultant—stands as a tested model for addressing the increasingly complex and demanding work of primary care. A strong PCP champion and PCP buy-in are crucial components to success. Shared accountability based on trust and respect among the patient, the PCP, the BHP, the psychiatric consultant, and the rest of the primary care team members can accomplish a mutual goal of better health for the patient, the family, and the community. These teams working together can do much to reach the quadruple aim of improved physical and behavioral health outcomes, exceptional patient experience, lower cost of care, and a renewed joy in work for all staff.

REFERENCES

Abe-Kim J, Takeuchi DT, Hong S, et al: Use of mental health-related services among immigrant and US-born Asian Americans: results from the National Latino and Asian American Study. Am J Public Health 97(1):91–98, 2007 17138905

Alegría M, Chatterji P, Wells K, et al: Disparity in depression treatment among racial and ethnic minority populations in the United States. Psychiatr Serv 59(11):1264–1272, 2008 18971402

Asarnow JR, Rozenman M, Wiblin J, et al: Integrated medical-behavioral care compared with usual primary care for child and adolescent behavioral health: a meta-analysis. JAMA Pediatr 169(10):929–937, 2015 26259143

Bodenheimer T, Sinsky C: From triple to quadruple aim: care of the patient requires care of the provider. Ann Fam Med 12(6):573–576, 2014 25384822

Bodenheimer TS, Smith MD: Primary care: proposed solutions to the physician shortage without training more physicians. Health Aff (Millwood) 32(11):1881–1886, 2013 24191075

Bodenheimer T, Ghorob A, Willard-Grace R, et al: The 10 building blocks of high-performing primary care. Ann Fam Med 12(2):166–171, 2014 24615313

Breslau J, Kendler KS, Su M, et al: Lifetime risk and persistence of psychiatric disorders across ethnic groups in the United States. Psychol Med 35(3):317–327, 2005 15841868

Collins PY: Using Collaborative Care to Reduce Racial and Ethnic Disparities in Mental Health Care. Presentation to National Advisory Mental Health Council, Na-tional Institute of Mental Health, September 13, 2012. Available at: https://www.nimh.nih.gov/about/advisory-boards-and-groups/namhc/index.shtml.

Colton CW, Manderscheid RW: Congruencies in increased mortality rates, years of potential life lost, and causes of death among public mental health clients in eight states. Prev Chronic Dis 3(2):A42, 2006 16539783

Cooper LA, Ghods Dinoso BK, Ford DE, et al: Comparative effectiveness of standard versus patient-centered collaborative care interventions for depression among African Americans in primary care settings: the BRIDGE Study. Health Serv Res 48(1):150–174, 2013 22716199

Davis TD, Deen T, Bryant-Bedell K, et al: Does minority racial-ethnic status moderate outcomes of collaborative care for depression? Psychiatr Serv 62(11):1282–1288, 2011 22211206

de Hert M, Correll CU, Bobes J, et al: Physical illness in patients with severe mental disorders. I. Prevalence, impact of medications and disparities in health care. World Psychiatry 10(1):52–77, 2011 21379357

Fortuna LR, Alegría M, Gao S: Retention in depression treatment among ethnic and racial minority groups in the United States. Depress Anxiety 27(5):485–494, 2010 20336808

Gilmer TP, Walker C, Johnson ED, et al: Improving treatment of depression among Latinos with diabetes using project Dulce and IMPACT. Diabetes Care 31(7):1324–1326, 2008 18356401

Gittell JH, Godfrey M, Thistlethwaite J: Interprofessional collaborative practice and relational coordination: improving healthcare through relationships. J Interprof Care 27(3):210–213, 2013 23082769

Goodman R: The Strengths and Difficulties Questionnaire: a research note. J Child Psychol Psychiatry 38(5):581–586, 1997 9255702

Guo T, Xiang YT, Xiao L, et al: Measurement-based care versus standard care for major depression: a randomized controlled trial with blind raters. Am J Psychiatry 172(10):1004–1013, 2015 26315978

Interian A, Martinez I, Rios L, et al: Adaptation of a motivational interviewing intervention to improve antidepressant adherence among Latinos. Cultur Divers Ethnic Minor Psychol 16(2):215–225, 2010 20438160

Johnson JG, Harris ES, Spitzer RL, Williams JB: The Patient Health Questionnaire for Adolescents: validation of an instrument for the assessment of mental disorders among adolescent primary care patients. J Adolesc Health 30(3):196–204, 2002 11869927

Kern J: Providing primary care in behavioral health settings, in Integrated Care: Working at the Interface of Primary Care and Behavioral Health. Edited by Raney LE. Arlington, VA, American Psychiatric Publishing, 2015, pp 169–191

Kessler RC, Berglund P, Demler O, et al: Lifetime prevalence and age-of-onset distributions of DSM-IV disorders in the National Comorbidity Survey Replication. Arch Gen Psychiatry 62(6):593–602, 2005 15939837

Knight JR, Sherritt L, Shrier LA, et al: Validity of the CRAFFT substance abuse screening test among adolescent clinic patients. Arch Pediatr Adolesc Med 156(6):607–614, 2002 12038895

Lee SY, Martins SS, Keyes KM, et al: Mental health service use by persons of Asian ancestry with DSM-IV mental disorders in the United States. Psychiatr Serv 62(10):1180–1186, 2011 21969644

Lester H, Tritter JQ, Sorohan H: Patients' and health professionals' views on primary care for people with serious mental illness: focus group study. BMJ 330(7500):1122, 2005 15843427

Levine S, Unützer J, Yip JY, et al: Physicians' satisfaction with a collaborative disease management program for late-life depression in primary care. Gen Hosp Psychiatry 27(6):383–391, 2005 16271652

Lorig KR, Sobel DS, Stewart AL, et al: Evidence suggesting that a chronic disease self-management program can improve health status while reducing hospitalization: a randomized trial. Med Care 37(1):5–14, 1999 10413387

Mauer B: Behavioral health/primary care integration: the four quadrant model and evidence based practices. February 2006. Available at: http://www.ibhp.org/uploads/file/Four%20Quadrant%20Model%20updated%202-06.pdf. Accessed September 21, 2016.

McCabe MP, Leas L: A qualitative study of primary health care access, barriers and satisfaction among people with mental illness. Psychol Health Med 13(3):303–312, 2008 18569898

Miranda J, Duan N, Sherbourne C, et al: Improving care for minorities: can quality improvement interventions improve care and outcomes for depressed minorities? Results of a randomized, controlled trial. Health Serv Res 38(2):613–630, 2003 12785564

Mitchell P, Wynia M, Golden R, et al: Core principles and values of effective team-based health care. National Academy of Sciences, Institute of Medicine 2012. Available at: https://www.nationalahec.org/pdfs/VSRT-Team-Based-Care-Principles-values.pdf. Accessed September 21, 2016.

Napoli M: Holistic health care for native women: an integrated model. Am J Public Health 92(10):1573–1575, 2002 12356594

Norfleet KR, Ratzliff AD, Chan YF, et al: The role of the integrated care psychiatrist in community settings: a survey of psychiatrists' perspectives. Psychiatr Serv 67(3):346–349, 2016 26695492

Ratzliff AD, Ni K, Chan YF, et al: A collaborative care approach to depression treatment for Asian Americans. Psychiatr Serv 64(5):487–490, 2013 23632577

Robins DL, Casagrande K, Barton M, et al: Validation of the Modified Checklist for Autism in Toddlers, Revised With Follow-Up (M-CHAT-R/F). Pediatrics 133(1):37–45, 2014 24366990

Samnaliev M, McGovern MP, Clark RE: Racial/ethnic disparities in mental health treatment in six Medicaid programs. J Health Care Poor Underserved 20(1):165–176, 2009 19202255

Scharf D, Eberhart N, Schmidt N, et al: Integrating primary care into community behavioral health settings: programs and early implementation experiences. Psychiatr Serv 64:660–665, 2013 23584674

Schonhaut L, Armijo I, Schönstedt M, et al: Validity of the ages and stages question-
naires in term and preterm infants. Pediatrics 131(5):e1468–e1474, 2013
23629619
Unützer J, Katon W, Callahan CM, et al; IMPACT Investigators. Improving Mood—
Promoting Access to Collaborative Treatment: collaborative care management
of late-life depression in the primary care setting: a randomized controlled trial.
JAMA 288(22):2836–2845, 2002 12472325
van Steenbergen-Weijenburg KM, van der Feltz-Cornelis CM, Horn EK, et al: Cost-
effectiveness of collaborative care for the treatment of major depressive disorder in primary care. A systematic review. BMC Health Serv Res 10(1):19, 2010
20082727
Wagner EH, Austin BT, Davis C, et al: Improving chronic illness care: translating evidence into action. Health Aff (Millwood) 20(6):64–78, 2001 11816692
Wagner EH, Austin B, Coleman C: It takes a region: creating a framework to improve
chronic disease care. California Healthcare Foundation. 2006. Available at:
http://www.improvingchroniccare.org/downloads/chcfreport.pdf. Accessed
September 21, 2016.
Wang PS, Berglund P, Olfson M, et al: Failure and delay in initial treatment contact
after first onset of mental disorders in the National Comorbidity Survey Replication. Arch Gen Psychiatry 62(6):603–613, 2005 15939838
Whitebird RR, Solberg LI, Jaeckels NA, et al: Effective implementation of collaborative care for depression: what is needed? Am J Manag Care 20(9):699–707, 2014
25365745
Wolraich ML, Lambert W, Doffing MA, et al: Psychometric properties of the
Vanderbilt ADHD diagnostic parent rating scale in a referred population. J Pediatr Psychol 28(8):559–567, 2003 14602846
Woltmann E, Grogan-Kaylor A, Perron B, et al: Comparative effectiveness of collaborative chronic care models for mental health conditions across primary, specialty, and behavioral health care settings: systematic review and meta-analysis.
Am J Psychiatry 169(8):790–804, 2012 22772364

CHAPTER 6

The Psychiatric Consultant

John Kern, M.D.

Lori E. Raney, M.D.

THE "ENGAGED" PSYCHIATRIC CONSULTANT

The behind-the-scenes psychiatric consultation is often referred to as the force multiplier of the Collaborative Care Model (CoCM), allowing leveraging of scarce psychiatric resources to provide effective care to more people in need. In their article on effective implementation of collaborative care, Whitebird et al. (2014) describe the importance of nine core factors that contribute to effectiveness (see Chapter 1, "Elements of Effective Design and Implementation," Table 1–6). The second highest-ranking factor was the presence of an "engaged psychiatrist," described as "responsive to the care manager and all patients, especially those that are not improving" (Whitebird et al. 2014), p. 701. When outcome is further divided into the two key categories of patient engagement and symptom remission (Patient Health Questionnaire–9 [PHQ-9] score < 5), the presence of the psychiatric consultant was vital to achieving remission at 6 months. The survey questions from the Whitebird study are listed in Table 6–1 and give a sense of the responses that led to how the authors interpreted "engaged."

ROLES OF THE PSYCHIATRIC CONSULTANT

Leadership

Much like the primary care provider (PCP) champion in Chapter 5, "The Primary Care Provider," an engaged psychiatric consultant leads through

---

TABLE 6–1. Psychiatrist survey questions

Do you or care managers meet routinely with the psychiatrist for the weekly 2-hour meetings?

Is the psychiatrist friendly and helpful with your review of patients in your caseload?

Does he or she give feedback, direction, or suggestions for both pharmacological and other therapeutic approaches to getting the patient to goal?

Do the psychiatrist and the primary care provider (PCP) ever connect?

If the PCP contacts the consulting psychiatrist in between the weekly sessions, does he or she typically get back to the PCP in a timely manner?

Has the psychiatrist done any other types of in-service or education sessions for your PCPs, your care managers, and/or care teams?

Do you have any concerns about the consulting psychiatrist working on your team?

Thanks to Nancy Jaeckels Kamp, R.N., for the contribution of her field notes from the study.

---

formal and informal means. Psychiatric consultants ensure maintenance of fidelity to the process, model collaborative relationships instead of hierarchy, manage resistance and conflict, create and sustain relationships with the essential individuals in the program, and persuade others about the value of collaborative care. In particular, they have the opportunity to straddle the medical and behavioral health worlds and leverage their credibility as a medical provider in persuading PCPs, who may initially be resistant to implementation for a host of reasons (see Chapter 5), to support culture change. This role of "boundary spanner" can be crucial to overcoming the cultural differences that exist in the historically siloed worlds of primary care and behavioral health.

One of the unique ways in which psychiatric consultants support the behavioral health provider (BHP) is in helping the BHP to manage PCP resistance or style. The psychiatric consultant can serve as a culture translator for BHPs in helping them learn how to function well in a medical setting and gain medical provider trust. The psychiatric consultant can also serve to support and nurture the BHP to help manage the stress encountered during a busy and unpredictable day in an unfamiliar environment. This support can help limit burnout and staff turnover of this essential team member, who serves as the boots on the ground and the eyes and ears for the psychiatric consultant. Checking in with the BHP at the beginning of the regularly scheduled caseload review can be a great way to start the meeting and let the BHP know he or she has support from the psychiatric consultant, who can be a sounding board for the issues the BHP is confronting. The psychiatric consultant's awareness about his or her relationship and interaction with the BHP is also important, because trust and confidence in the BHP's skill level is necessary, and if such trust is lacking, this issue should be openly addressed. Finally, the psychiatric consultant serves to make sure the voice of the BHP is heard. It may be a bit intimidating for BHPs to be surrounded by medical doctors, in particular, and it is important to ensure their unique perspective is valued.

Physical presence in the clinic is an important way of getting to know the team and building trust, in particular with the PCPs. However, it is not always possible in every setting because of the consultant's location, which may be in a distant site. An on-site visit or in-person training during team development and before launching the model can help initial relationship building with the entire team. Following this on-site presence, there is an opportunity for continued relationship formation and team building during times of teleconferencing or other electronic communication. The success of teleconferencing for off-site education and case-based learning programs such as Project ECHO (Extension for Community Healthcare Outcomes, http://echo.unm.edu) have emphasized the importance of paying close attention to relationships in every meeting and setting aside time for check-in and discussion of team dynamics (see Chapter 3, "Team Development and Culture").

"Family docs build long-term trusting relationships with their patients and would not refer a patient to someone they do not trust or would not go to themselves. It needs to feel like a caring [and] trusting relationship with the psychiatric consultant first and not like it is just transactional."—*C.K., family medicine physician, Indianapolis, Indiana*

Consultation: Extending Psychiatric Expertise to Larger Populations

The psychiatric consultant provides indirect and direct consultation. Many PCPs are at first disappointed to learn that the psychiatric provider will not be directly seeing patients on-site in a traditional co-located referral format and may express frustration because they may have anxiety about addressing behavioral health conditions in their practice. Through education and team development, both the organizational leaders and the psychiatric consultant can begin to shift provider expectations of the role of psychiatric consultation and the advantages over traditional referral. The goal is to provide straightforward care for straightforward problems in the most efficient manner, reserving direct psychiatric provider time for the complicated cases that have not responded.

The CoCM employs minimal face-to-face contact between the patient and psychiatric consultant and substitutes a proactive primary care team, a well-defined structure of screening and protocols providing evidence-based interventions, registry tracking with persistent monitoring, and access to the expertise of the psychiatric consultant for review of more challenging cases. From the point of view of the psychiatric provider, this limitation of face-to-face contact may be undesirable because it seems contrary to the reason for entering the field in the first place: interacting with patients. If one imagined a psychiatric workplace in which there was never any direct interaction with patients, it would probably be difficult to find clinicians to work there, even if it was particularly successful at improving the psychiatric outcomes of patients. And yet, psychiatrists who work in CoCM settings almost universally enjoy it (Norfleet et al. 2016). The relationships with coworkers are sustaining, and the opportunity to be exposed to a large number of clinical stories provides real growth for psychiatric consultants who take the work seriously and pay attention to the clinical scenarios to which they are exposed. Psychiatric consultants are also exposed to a wide variety of unfamiliar subject areas for consultation, which provide opportunities for stretching their skill set and significant opportunities for professional learning.

Indirect Consultation

Indirect consultation is the force multiplier for the CoCM, allowing more patients to benefit from psychiatric expertise than is possible when treating each patient individually. Indirect consultation includes curbside consultation immediately available to the primary care team and regularly scheduled caseload reviews for additional input for patients who are not progressing in treatment. This behind-the-scenes activity, where the psychiatric consultant can provide input on many more patients than if all were seen (or agreed to be seen), can address the national shortage of psychiatric expertise by as much as an order of magnitude. However, reimbursement for this indirect activity is a significant barrier to wider implementation of CoCM in a fee-for-service environment (see Chapter 8, "Financing Integrated Care") because these services that are proven to be effective cannot be coded, billed, or reimbursed in the traditional health care model.

Some psychiatric consultants may be initially concerned about liability when providing recommendations for patients they have not directly examined (Lambert and Bland 2015), and this concern may limit their willingness to participate in these teams. Currently, the legal precedent for traditional curbside consultation does not meet the level of engagement necessary to define a doctor-patient relationship. Historically in these situations, liability is felt to be minimal. In the CoCM, where the clinical involvement exceeds that of the typical curbside relationship, the liability exposure of the psychiatric consultant remains unclear. It would be reasonable to assume that it is greater than traditional indirect consultation. However, the CoCM provides better care than the typical standard of care in the primary care setting, and this level of care may mitigate some of the liability. To date there are no cases of successful litigation against a consulting psychiatric provider on a collaborative care team. Malpractice insurance carriers are frequently unfamiliar with the case law and literature in this area and may unnecessarily recommend that psychiatric consultants avoid participating on these teams. A very useful resource, "Risk Management and Liability Issues in Integrated Care Models," was prepared by the American Psychiatric Association and can be shared with a carrier (www.psychiatry.org/psychiatrists/search-directories-databases/library-and-archive/resource documents) and reviewed for details.

Curbside consultation

The most frequent task of many psychiatric consultants is the curbside consultation with the PCP or the BHP, which does not include direct evaluation as mentioned earlier. The most common reasons for consultation are requests for medication recommendations and diagnostic clarification for mood, anxiety, and substance use disorders as illustrated in Figure 6–1 (Norfleet et al. 2016). Consultations can occur via the phone, texting, e-mail, or tasking in an electronic health record. Electronic consultation platforms have been developed and have demonstrated a reduction in referrals to specialists (Olayiwola et al. 2016). This method could be adapted to the psychiatric consultation as long as quick access can be arranged. An organized approach to the curbside consultation is presented in the section "The 'Nicely DONE' Mnemonic" later in this chapter.

Curbside consultation provides a mechanism for case-based learning that takes the PCP and BHP concerns and applies immediate guidance for them to act on. This process is much more active than traditional educational experiences, which tend to be done through a more passive approach (e.g., attending lectures). This more dynamic method is thought to be best suited for adult learners (Knowles 1984), and most psychiatric consultants witness this

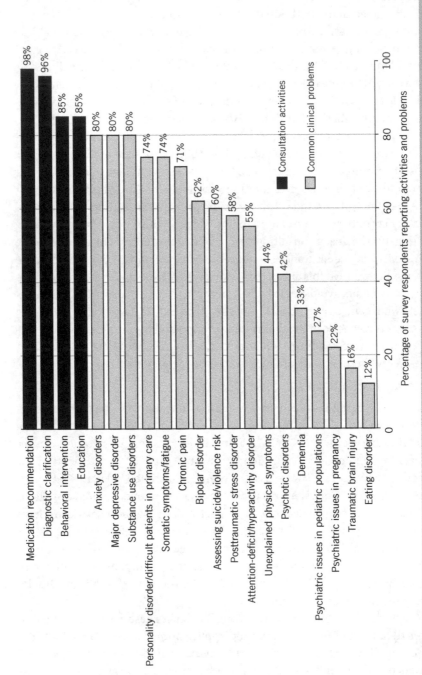

FIGURE 6–1. Consultation activities and common clinical problems reported by psychiatrists in integrated care.

Source. Adapted from Norfleet KR, Ratzliff AD, Chan YF, et al.: "The Role of the Integrated Care Psychiatrist in Community Settings: A Survey of Psychiatrists' Perspectives." *Psychiatric Services* 67(3):346–349, 2016. Copyright © 2016 American Psychiatric Association. Used with permission.

growth in knowledge occurring as they are asked more difficult questions by the PCP and BHP over time. In addition, this change in practice behavior has demonstrated results in the form of improved outcomes confirmed by measurement tools such as the PHQ-9 for depression.

Some concerns have been raised that collaborative care is overly medication focused. Resistance to the notion of an overly medicalized approach to behavioral health care seems highly appropriate. The application of the tools of psychiatric practice to the care of medical patients both humanizes the care of those patients and extends the reach of psychiatric expertise to patients who are unable or afraid to seek out this care in the mental health system as presently available. The antidote to practicing in an overly medicalized way is, of course, not to succumb to the pressure to see every patient as a problem to be medicated, and to continue to remain familiar with the aspects of personal experience and the scope of psychological treatment for the problems that patients present. Some consults will quickly raise questions about the need for social or behavioral interventions. Psychiatric consultants can bring this perspective and share it repeatedly with PCPs, who in turn expand their understanding of patients and help themselves to begin thinking about behavioral health treatment in a more evidence-based and expansive manner. This perspective also serves to support and validate the role of the BHP, who works exclusively in the realm of behavior change and who addresses the psychosocial barriers to health. An effective psychiatric consultant should anticipate the need to remind colleagues on a daily basis of the importance of behavioral approaches.

One may wonder how definitive psychiatric diagnosis can be with a comparatively brief contact with a BHP, even with backup psychiatric consultation. The primary care clinical setting offers a host of unexpected advantages in this regard. There are a number of pieces of information and support available to the treatment teams that are not always readily available to the individual psychiatric practitioner. For example, PCPs often have histories and relationships with these patients, know their families and social circumstances, and certainly know their medical histories, medication lists, and prior treatment. The clinic's behavioral health protocol may include standardized assessment of depression, anxiety, substance abuse, and in some settings such things as signs of posttraumatic stress disorder. This backdrop results in quite a bit of information being available to the team before even beginning the interview.

In primary care settings, there are many kinds of clinical scenarios that are treated presumptively without a definitive diagnosis, for example, straightforward urinary tract infections or uncomplicated allergy symptoms. Commonly encountered psychiatric scenarios resemble these primary care examples, such as new-onset panic attacks, sleep problems, and straightforward depressive episodes without bipolar or psychotic complications. It is rational to deal with these presumptively, without requiring a long list of rule outs to be satisfied first. It is also sensible to make sure that all parties involved—patient, PCP, BHP, and family—understand the iterative process of establishing a definitive diagnosis. Treatment can happen in the primary care setting in the presence of continuing communication, whether, for example, in ongoing PCP visits, behavioral health visits, or telephone calls. The primary care infrastructure supports rapid and effective communication between patients and treaters much more than does the standard specialty behavioral health treatment model, not to mention how much simpler it is to get needed laboratory studies or even an urgent appointment for a clinical contact in primary care.

Psychiatric consultants have found that it can take some time to get used to the curbside consultation process, but once established and running smoothly, it can be a very rewarding and novel experience. Time demands are usually not extravagant. PCPs and BHPs are typically grateful for the psychiatric consultant's willingness to be interrupted and therefore are usually respectful of the time. In addition, the caseload-focused registry review (discussed in the next subsection) provides an ongoing opportunity to measure the effect of the curbside experience and alleviate concerns about not knowing the outcome of the consultation.

"Initially I was anxious about consulting on patients I have not personally examined. My experience has been it is very freeing to be able to provide some care without the intensity of forming relationships with every patient I see."—*Psychiatric consultant, California*

Caseload-focused registry review

Regularly scheduled review of the registry by the psychiatric consultant for each BHP's caseload is a crucial process that helps identify patients who are not progressing as expected or engaging in treatment, and allows for additional treatment recommendations to be made and discussed with the BHP and relayed to the PCP if necessary. This classic application of population health allows providers to see what is happening, and not happening, with patients and intervene to provide effective care. The registry can be reviewed off-site via phone or teleconferencing, as long as each party has access to the registry and preferably at least one party has access to the electronic health record of the patients prioritized for review at that session.

The capacity for collaborative care to improve outcomes is found in this systematic approach, most notably the functions of regular structured assessment, timely response to suboptimal treatment response, and outreach to patients who are not engaged in regular treatment. This approach is what permits the relatively thin, or even extremely thin, quantity of psychiatric consultation time to be used efficiently to answer the more difficult questions and to figure out when something just doesn't sound right. This attention to continually measuring outcomes and assisting the PCP and BHP in adjusting treatment if targets are not being met, supported by data tracked in the registry, is at the heart of efforts to drive outcomes toward remission. And it is an engaged psychiatric consultant who can oversee this process by consistently urging the team to use the registry and by assisting in treatment planning for a subset of patients who are not progressing. Figure 6–2 reports the findings of a study that reveals the value of psychiatric consultation between weeks 8 and 12 for patients who are not improving, demonstrating they had a greater likelihood of improvement by week 24 (Bao et al. 2016).

Some psychiatric consultants may choose to document their recommendations from the caseload review and include them as a note or addendum in the patients' electronic health records, whereas others may choose to provide advice verbally, which is then recorded by the BHP and relayed to the PCP. If a note is written, it is important to include a disclaimer that the patient has not been evaluated directly and to document the discussion with the BHP and any records reviewed. New physician codes under review by the Centers for Medicare and Medicaid Services may require written notes and documentation of which patients were reviewed when consultation was provided in order to receive reimbursement for the psychiatric consultant's efforts (for more details see Chapter 7, "Policy and Regulatory Environment"). Closing the loop at a later time by further review allows the consultant to see if the PCP implemented the recommendations and what outcomes were achieved.

The registry review allows the team to see the population health impact of their services. Providers often are not aware of the influence their practice is having on the population health of their patients and of the potential value of this practice to the overall health system. They need to be reminded of this impact, as they tend to focus on the everyday difficulties of the work and not to experience the reward of its effectiveness on the greater level.

Data from the registry can be aggregated and used in varying ways, such as determining a clinic's overall performance, comparing the tasks provided by individual staff members to see if they meet guidelines, discovering trends that may lead to providing additional education, or recognizing there are care gaps that need remediation. The importance of close attention to the accuracy and timely recording of data in the registry cannot be stressed

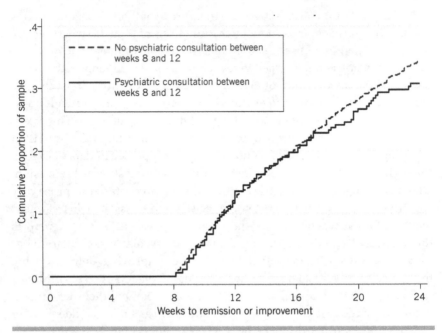

FIGURE 6–2.   Effect of psychiatric consultation between weeks 8 and 12.

Note.   Time to first clinically significant improvement in depression among patients in a collaborative care model, by psychiatric consultation between weeks 8 and 12 among patients not achieving improvement by week 8.
Source.   Reprinted from Bao Y, Druss BG, Jung HY, et al.: "Unpacking Collaborative Care for Depression: Examining Two Essential Tasks for Implementation." *Psychiatric Services* 67(4):418–424, 2016. Copyright © 2016 American Psychiatric Association. Used with permission.

enough, and there is a high probability that this information will be used to inform payers and accrediting bodies of a clinic's progress. The psychiatric consultant can serve as a guardian of this process during the regularly scheduled reviews to make sure the registry is well maintained, accurate, and up-to-date.

Direct Consultation

Direct consultation is infrequent, occurring in only 5%–7% of patients in the initial Improving Mood—Promoting Access to Collaborative Treatment (IMPACT) study (Unützer et al. 2002). However, there are occasionally circumstances when select patients who are not making progress may benefit from one or two brief visits with the psychiatric consultant to sort out more complex concerns and thus to preclude referral to specialty care. Direct consultation can be done face-to-face or by teleconferencing, depending on clinic resources and the availability of the psychiatric consultant. Teleconferencing helps to reduce the time lost to lengthy commutes, allowing more direct service to be provided, and should be considered along with some occasional on-site visits to help the psychiatric consultant form relationships with the team. It is important the BHP act as the gatekeeper to the consultant's time to prevent direct referral by PCPs who may wish to circumvent the stepped care process for various reasons, including their discomfort in treating mental health and substance use conditions. Some sites may have on-site traditional psychiatric practices where referral can eventually be made if ongoing specialty behavioral health care is deemed the appropriate next step in treatment. The ability to use the indirect services of the psychiatric consultant can help manage the flow to specialty services and to ensure patients with mild to moderate disorders are being treated by the PCP and BHP. Of course, the consultant and the on-site traditional psychiatric provider could be the same individual. This situation would need to be managed carefully to prevent a slippery slope toward co-location, because the pressure from PCPs to have the psychiatric provider directly care for these patients can be intense. One approach could be to establish a protocol to evaluate patients once or twice in consultation with prompt referral back to the PCP. Patients who are referred for specialty care should also be accepted back to the primary care setting once they become sufficiently stable for this step down in level of management. This approach should be discussed with the PCP and BHP ahead of time to avoid confusion and conflict. This frees up the psychiatric providers in specialty behavioral health to have greater capacity and improves access for patients with more severe illness who need that level of care (see the section "The Continuum of Collaborative Services and Cycle of Patients Within This System of Care" in Chapter 1).

This process of cycling through as appropriate can help maintain access to care and sufficient distribution of limited hours of psychiatric expertise in a given organization. The following quotation shows how one psychiatric consultant can support several BHP caseloads and provide expert input to literally hundreds of patients at a time, delivering at least an order of magnitude of increased capacity.

"At present, I am paid for 6 hours per week (0.15 FTE) to provide consultative support to five BHPs, who provide approximately 500 encounters per month, and coverage of more than 35,000 lives in two primary care systems. Over the more than 7 years I have been doing this, I have documented about 5,000 phone or in-person consultations. This adds up to about five calls per day, averaging 3.6 minutes per call. This is an extraordinary scaling up of psychiatric expertise over a big population, with a use of psychiatric time that is relatively minimal."—*Psychiatric consultant, Indiana*

Educator

Another core task of the psychiatric consultant is that of continuously providing education for the team, which can take the form of embedding information in the informal consultations mentioned earlier. Every consultation should function as a learning experience and present an opportunity to teach. This serves as a mechanism to provide case-based learning to increase knowledge that can be applied to current and future situations. Education can also be provided through presentations at team meetings on subjects of interest to providers, the distribution of relevant articles, and the sharing of treatment algorithms and information on useful Web sites or conferences. The breadth and depth of psychiatric education provides an extensive pool of valuable information. The primary goal in the role of educator is to increase the competence and confidence of the team to move forward in the "sweet spot" of capability in the primary care setting: treating mild to moderate mental illnesses in a stepped care manner that measures progress along the way, treats to defined targets, and refers patients who need additional services to specialty behavioral health care.

"Just come and talk about something. It's more interesting than another lecture on asthma."—*Primary care provider to the psychiatric consultant, Indiana*

Patients present in a primary care clinic with more than just depression and anxiety, and it is necessary for the psychiatric consultant to be prepared to offer recommendations on a variety of conditions and populations that may expand the consultant's usual practice or extend past the traditional case base. This adaptability by the psychiatric consultant allows access to mental health and substance abuse services for many people who could not or would not otherwise have accessed them. Such adaptability creates challenges for all involved to care for conditions for which the team may have less expertise. Assessing progress for these patients is also usually more difficult, because there is often not a measure of response to treatment for attention-deficit/hyperactivity disorder (ADHD) or for bipolar disorder that is as straightforward and tested as the PHQ-9 is for depression. These difficulties require the psychiatric consultant to take steps to expand his or her scope of expertise into areas such as pediatric psychopharmacology (for adult psychiatric consultants) or substance use disorders. It is important to gain additional knowledge in some areas and to have personal educational resources for times when this is needed. The consultant needs to seek information, education, and training in order to provide the best possible support to the patient and the clinical team—in other words, to broaden his or her expertise.

"When I began doing this work, I had never diagnosed or treated ADHD in an adult or a child—a shortcoming of my professional development, it turned out. At first, I would inform my consultees that this just wasn't part of my toolkit, but I quickly learned the general rule for the primary care psychiatric consultant that nothing is not part of your toolkit, at least not for long. So I read up, took a course, and consulted my child psychiatric colleagues, and began at least to have a basic understanding of how to approach these problems. One might say that a basic understanding is less than what our patients deserve. On the other hand, the actual situation on the ground is usually that even this is more than presently is available to patients. I believe that a basic understanding, underpinned by other clinical experience of some degree of applicability, and a relatively hard-headed insistence on following the dictates of the medical evidence, is a good first step in the direction of a more sophisticated understanding and practice."—*Psychiatric consultant, Indiana*

Another educational task is providing protocols for the PCP and BHP to follow, and designing these can be a team effort that helps relieve tension around situations such as suicidality or substance use concerns. Box 6–1 provides an example of a psychiatric consultant developing a policy on benzodiazepine use in a primary care setting.

Box 6–1. Policy Example: Use of benzodiazepines

"This has been a popular policy with primary care providers, who grow cynical and fatigued by frequent requests for these medications that they view as inappropriate. In general the policy is that we do not prescribe benzodiazepines at all, except for very rare exceptions, and for weaning off patients who have presented with significant benzodiazepine doses. This policy is presented early on by the PCPs to the patients to prevent any confusion or misunderstanding with the BHP. Weaning will be done carefully over several weeks or even months for patients who have a credible history, and rather more quickly, primarily to avoid medical morbidity, in patients who may have been using these medications inappropriately."—*John Kern, M.D., Chief Medical Officer, Regional Mental Health Center, Merrillville, Indiana*

Basic principles:

- Benzodiazepines have a limited role in the management of anxiety disorders.
- Selective serotonin reuptake inhibitors (SSRIs) and behavioral measures are first-line treatments.
- Often anxiety is a presenting symptom of other mental health conditions.
- Risk of substance abuse is significant in the population.

Agreement about the obligation to change culture in the organization and community in the way we address the following psychiatric issues:

- Risk of controlled substances.
- Role of nonmedication treatment.
- Identifying substance abuse in patients.

Recommendations:

- Avoid use of benzodiazepines as first-line treatment of anxiety, agitation, and insomnia.
- Become familiar with and encourage use of sleep hygiene education and techniques. A good sleep history can be done in a few minutes.
- Taper dosage in clients who present with benzodiazepine use; even if they have taken the medication for many years, this does not necessarily make it a good idea.
- If tapering, set a schedule and do not permit "early fills" of medications.
- Use BHP as resource if needed.
- Use the Prescription Drug Monitoring Program to limit clinic shopping.

THE "NICELY DONE" MNEMONIC

Originally discussed in Raney (2015), a thorough and efficient curbside consultation can be broken down into a series of specific components. A useful approach for remembering these components can be found in the mnemonic "Nicely DONE."

- **Nicely:** Building mutual trust and rapport
- **D: Diagnosis:** establish a provisional diagnosis in order to move forward
- **O: Offer** concise feedback and suggestions
- **N: Next** steps and "if-then" scenarios
- **E: Education:** every consult presents an opportunity to teach

This simple reminder of the core tasks and interpersonal approach serves as a guide to psychiatric consultants of the content expertise, interpersonal competencies, and support they need to deliver in order to enhance the competence and capacity of the primary care–based team.

Nicely: Building Mutual Trust and Rapport

Historically, psychiatrists in particular have struggled with maintaining collegial relationships with other medical providers, who might remember psychiatric providers not returning their calls, feel that their referrals end up in a "black hole," or sense an unwillingness on the part of psychiatrists to share information. Thus psychiatrists need to take special care during the consultation process to handle these communication issues in a respectful and courteous manner. "Nicely" refers to the steps taken that ensure the process leads to successfully building trusting relationships that reassure the BHP and PCP that they are well supported in moving forward with treatment that they may feel is outside their scope of practice. Box 6–2 provides examples that demonstrate some core features of this collegial process.

Box 6–2. The Collegial Process

Maintain a welcoming tone

- "How can I help you?"
- "How's it going?
- "No need to apologize for the call. I'm here to help you."

Be readily accessible

- Answer a call immediately if possible.
- If not able to answer immediately, then strive for within 2 hours.
- Be flexible in the mode of communication and adapt to what best suits the primary care–based team (e.g., phone, text, e-mail, messaging and/or tasking in electronic medical record, e-consult).

Offer praise for things they have already done well

- "It's good you tried an SSRI first."
- "Getting a repeat PHQ-9 was really helpful."
- "I'm glad you thought to get the thyroid function test."

Avoid critical statements

- PCPs may already think they have done something wrong and this may be the reason they are calling.
- The tone of voice used in asking something like "Why did you choose to do that?" can sound either critical or curious to the person on the other end of the line.

Be respectful

- What PCPs are doing is important and may be anxiety provoking.
- Demonstrate that you understand the seriousness of what is occurring and approach the issue appropriately.

D: Diagnosis: Establish a Provisional Diagnosis in Order to Move Forward

- **Determine the chief complaint quickly.** You will not necessarily have all the information—decide what is a good balance and move forward.
- **Assess provider comfort level and abilities** (e.g., "Are you familiar with augmentation in the treatment of depression?"; "How comfortable are you with the diagnosis of bipolar disorder?").
- **Gather additional pertinent information.** There may be things that have been missed, particularly in areas such as a history of trauma, substance use, or safety.

- **Discuss the differential diagnosis and make a provisional diagnosis to move forward.** PCPs are often comfortable with the concept of more than one possible diagnosis. Let them know what you think they should concentrate on first.

O: Offer Concise Feedback and Suggestions

Respect time constraints

- Both of you are busy (e.g., "Do you have time to discuss this further or do you need to go?").
- Avoid a lengthy musing of all that could be going on with the patient and stick to what is pertinent at that moment.

Offer evidence-based pharmacological and nonpharmacological suggestions

- Know the evidence-based medication guidelines—don't just suggest your favorite medications.
- PCPs may have more comfort and familiarity with something that is equivalent to what you have suggested (e.g., "If you're more familiar with sertraline, it's OK to start there instead of with the citalopram I recommended").
- Know the evidence-based brief interventions commonly used in primary care by BHPs and recommend changes in approach if warranted.
- Offer a titration plan for medications if needed.
- Make sure to review pertinent side effects.

Avoid excessive psychiatric jargon

- It's all right to introduce some of the language of behavioral health, and PCPs are generally interested in learning (e.g., "We call that splitting, and I'll make sure to discuss this in our next team meeting so that everyone understands how to deal with the situation next time, OK?"), but avoid going overboard.

Recommend measurement and screening tools

- "Has the PHQ-9 been repeated? If not, I recommend that to help you measure this patient's response to treatment."

- "The GAD-7 [Generalized Anxiety Disorder 7-item scale] is a nice way of tracking anxiety symptoms. Do you have a copy there or would you like me to send you one?"

Tailor advice to local resources

- There is little use in recommending a treatment modality or service, such as dialectical behavioral therapy or partial hospitalization, if you know this isn't available locally (e.g., "I would usually recommend aripiprazole in a presentation like this, but with your limited formulary let's try risperidone instead").
- Work with the BHP to understand what is available so you are prepared to offer actionable advice.

N: Next Steps and "If-Then" Scenarios

Offer alternative strategies if plan A doesn't work

- "I recommend you start with sertraline and if this doesn't work, I suggest switching to a different class of antidepressants and try a serotonin norepinephrine reuptake inhibitor (SNRI) such as venlafaxine next."
- "Bupropion is a good first choice in this case since she is trying to quit smoking, but if it makes her anxious, you can switch to fluoxetine given her history of medication trials."

Summarize plan before ending the call

- Keep the summary short and concise.
- A few bullet points quickly highlights the plan.

Encourage provider to call back if needed

- "If you have any concerns, please do not hesitate to call me."
- "Give me a call and let me know how it goes."

E: Education: Every Consult Presents an Opportunity to Teach

Tactfully embed education into the consultation.

- Don't make it into a lecture.
- Lengthy explanations take up valuable time and might convey that you don't think the listener knows anything about appropriate treatment.

Build the provider's confidence and capacity to manage psychiatric disorders.

- Every contact with a BHP or PCP can and should include an explanation for why a specific consultative recommendation is being made. If they already knew what to do, they probably wouldn't have called in the first place.
  — "The reason I recommended lithium is because most of his symptoms fall in the category of mania, and this is a good treatment for this type of bipolar disorder."
  — "I suggest you try fluoxetine since this worked for her mother, and from a genetic standpoint it may work for her too."
- As people who teach know, having to explain yourself creates a desire to know the subject matter more completely—this is a potent stimulus to learning for the psychiatric consultant.

Be brief—less than a minute usually.

- You can tuck a kernel of education quickly into a consultation, as demonstrated above.
- Learning is an iterative process, and there may be more time in a formal didactic to think again about a case.

Example Consultations Using the Nicely DONE Mnemonic

The case example and following excerpts of responses from the psychiatric consultant delineate each of the principles outlined for Nicely DONE.

Case Example

A 43-year-old female with a history of posttraumatic stress disorder and major depression presents to her PCP for follow-up. The PCP prescribed citalopram 20 mg last month, and the patient experienced facial swelling that led to discontinuation of the medication for a presumed allergic reaction. The PCP selected bupropion as the next medication, and the BHP is reporting that the patient called today and is experiencing marked agitation, anger outbursts, and heightened anxiety. The patient has not been sleeping well, and this worsened with the initiation of bupropion. The patient has been working with the BHP on relaxation techniques and behavioral activation. Her initial PHQ-9 score was 16, and today over the phone her score was 18. The PCP is requesting consultation to see if the patient should be started on quetiapine for a presumed diagnosis of bipolar disorder due to the reaction to bupropion and to help with her sleep difficulties.

Excerpts: Psychiatric Consultant Response to PCP in Case Example

Nicely: "Hi, Mark. How are things going at the clinic? How can I help you today?"

D: "Is there a history of bipolar disorder? Any symptoms of mania? Is she using any substances such as alcohol or marijuana? Is there any relevant medical history I should know about?"

O: "Based on what you told me it sounds like she is pretty anxious and had an increase in symptoms on the bupropion. At this time it does not sound like bipolar disorder because I am not hearing there are any symptoms of mania, but we'll keep a close watch on this as we move forward. I suggest you try another SSRI such as sertraline or fluoxetine since she's only tried citalopram in the past. She's just started working with the BHP with some therapeutic interventions, and she may get some symptom relief as that progresses too. We'll track her carefully and repeat her PHQ-9 several times over the next month and see how she responds. Trazodone 50–100 mg for sleep is fine for now. I would not prescribe quetiapine at this point."

N: "If she does not experience improvement on the new medication I suggest you try an SNRI such as venlafaxine next. If she has any clear symptoms of bipolar disorder, you can consider a mood stabilizer instead. Give me a call if that occurs and I will walk you through that process if you need my help."

E: "The reason I don't think she has bipolar disorder is there's no family history and no prior history. An important distinction between bipolar and unipolar depression is the presence of symptoms of mania, and I'm not hearing she has experienced any euphoric or grandiose symptoms. It seems she's more irritated than anything, and this is a somewhat pervasive symptom for her, maybe related to her trauma. We'll get this sorted out as the team gets to know her over time. Also, I typically recommend a trial of two SSRIs before moving to another class of antidepressants. It is cleaner to go with a medication that has a single mechanism of action. Bupropion is in its own class and that didn't work out for her, so the SNRIs would be next, and they have a dual action. Please give me a call if you have any questions or concerns."

PERSONAL OPPORTUNITIES IN COLLABORATIVE CARE

The unique experiences and learning opportunities presented while working in a collaborative care setting can enhance everyday psychiatric practice. These include exposure to a lot of cases, new perspectives on the ability to diagnose and treat, expansion of clinical competence, and opportunities for using screening and measurement tools. In addition, there is not only the experience of learning what one can contribute in encounters with PCPs and BHPs, but also the humbling experience of what one can learn. The consultant role can shift the identity of psychiatric providers, who will find that they are not always the expert and instead will benefit from a willingness to learn from others. A survey of psychiatric consultants from across the country looked at their experiences working in the CoCM. By far, their experiences were very positive and they benefited from having the opportunities to perform in the many roles that are described in this chapter (Norfleet et al. 2016).

THE IDEAL PSYCHIATRIC CONSULTANT

Engaged psychiatric consultants have many qualities that make them not only personally successful on the collaborative care team but also lead to better outcomes as demonstrated in Whitebird et al. (2014). This set of attributes (Table 6–2) is important to the success of the integration efforts of collaborative care teams, and close attention should be paid when hiring individuals for the job of psychiatric consultant on integrated teams.

FUTURE DIRECTIONS IN PSYCHIATRIC CONSULTATION

The use of technology is rapidly expanding the way health care is delivered, and there soon may be an increasing use of mobile apps, wearable devices, and other approaches that allow patients to co-manage their conditions. It is easy enough to imagine the day when providers can prompt patients to repeat a PHQ-9 on their wristwatch and remind them of a task they identified in a session of behavioral activation. This process can serve as a treatment extender for the BHP, PCP, and psychiatric consultant. The use of technology in this way will allow more frequent contact with patients, which has demonstrated benefit in improving outcomes (Bao et al. 2016). Expanding

TABLE 6–2. Personal attributes of an ideal psychiatric consultant

Friendly and outgoing personality works best

Flexible and OK with unexpected events

Adaptable to populations outside of expertise and the needs of the
primary care clinic

Available and willing to tolerate interruptions

Able to manage liability concerns about informal consultation

Enjoys teaching and learning

Appreciates being part of a team

Willing to lead—formally or informally

the clinical team through the use of technology allows improved access to behavioral health services and potential cost savings.

Providing collaborative care in remote areas without access to BHPs or psychiatric consultants is also a future possibility. Programs that centralize the collaborative care team in an academic or other setting can provide behavioral health "telehubs" (Fortney et al. 2013; see Chapter 1) where the BHP could be available via "e-handoff" on a tablet and the psychiatric consultant continues to be available by phone, teleconferencing, or even an in-home session. Data collected electronically can be centralized and analyzed, allowing treatment changes and outreach to occur in a less resource-intensive way than is currently available. Countries with few psychiatric providers could employ collaborative care teams from outside their borders, widening the international reach of expertise. An openness to these changes by psychiatric consultants will be important to continuing the goal of addressing the burden of mental health and substance abuse conditions. A future where the needs of the global community can be met, without the expectation that more human resources will necessarily be available, may be within our reach.

REFERENCES

Bao Y, Druss BG, Jung HY, et al: Unpacking collaborative care for depression: examining two essential tasks for implementation. Psychiatr Serv 67(4):418–424, 2016 26567934

Fortney JC, Pyne JM, Mouden SB, et al: Practice-based versus telemedicine-based collaborative care for depression in rural Federally Qualified Health Centers: a pragmatic randomized comparative effectiveness trial. Am J Psychiatry 170(4):414–425, 2013 23429924

Knowles M: The Adult Learner: A Neglected Species, 3rd Edition. Houston, TX, Gulf Publishing, 1984

Lambert L, Bland A: Risk management and liability issues in integrated care, in Integrated Care: Working at the Interface of Primary Care and Behavioral Health. Edited by Raney LE. Arlington, VA, American Psychiatric Publishing, 2015, pp 91–111

Norfleet KR, Ratzliff AD, Chan YF, et al: The role of the integrated care psychiatrist in community settings: a survey of psychiatrists' perspectives. Psychiatr Serv 67(3):346–349, 2016 26695492

Olayiwola JN, Anderson D, Jepeal N, et al: Electronic consultations to improve the primary care–specialty care interface for cardiology in the medically underserved: a cluster randomized controlled trial. Ann Fam Med 14(2):133–140, 2016 26951588

Raney LE: Integrating primary care and behavioral health: the role of the psychiatrist in the collaborative care model. Am J Psychiatry 172(8):721–728, 2015 26234599

Unützer J, Katon W, Callahan CM, et al; IMPACT Investigators. Improving Mood—Promoting Access to Collaborative Treatment: collaborative care management of late-life depression in the primary care setting: a randomized controlled trial. JAMA 288(22):2836–2845, 2002 12472325

Whitebird RR, Solberg LI, Jaeckels NA, et al: Effective implementation of collaborative care for depression: what is needed? Am J Manag Care 20(9):699–707, 2014 25365745

Part III

Operational Considerations

CHAPTER 7

Policy and Regulatory Environment

Ron Manderscheid, Ph.D.

Most assuredly, integration of somatic and behavioral health care represents the principal system reform issue facing behavioral health care at present. Depending on the individual's vantage point in the system, the view of progress and longevity of integration is quite different. For individuals engaged at the policy level, implementation of integration is far behind, whereas those on the ground delivering care often feel that practice is ahead of policy. In reality, national policy around system integration has been under development for almost three decades, whereas the practice of integration remains in its infancy, varying widely from community to community. How and why do these disconnects occur? This chapter examines the interplay between policy and practice transformation in relationship to integration and will explore the evolution of policy and practice, the role policy has played in shaping practice models, and what conditions influence practice lagging behind policy or policy lagging behind practice.

KEY CONCEPTS

Integrated care is the joint availability of mental health, substance use, and primary health care for a single patient. In its simplest form, this may represent nothing more complex than to provide behavioral health care and then refer the patient to another provider for needed primary care, or the reverse. The focus of this book is the more complex model of collaborative care, with integration occurring through a fully integrated treatment team that includes behavioral health and primary care providers. Specifically, this team may include primary care providers, nurses, a psychologist or social worker, a psychiatric consultant, and, in a growing number of settings, a peer support worker and other team members who may assist patients in getting their social services needs met.

Fundamentally, the goal of integrated care is whole person care that considers all of the health care needs of the patient by bringing the head and the body together. The reason for doing this is very clear: behavioral and physical health problems very frequently co-occur. As a classic example, depression co-occurs with cardiovascular disease (17% of cases), cerebrovascular disease (23%), and diabetes (27%), and recent data suggest that 70% of office visits that recorded a depression diagnosis also recorded the presence of a co-occurring chronic physical health condition (Jolles et al. 2015). There is also the patient experience to consider, in that individuals receive care that is coordinated and holistic rather than having to serve as the connector between a set of providers that do not share information.

Policy is the formal national policy that has been institutionalized through legislation and the cascading changes subsequently pushed down to states and regional entities. A full treatment of how national policy is developed and implemented is beyond the scope of this chapter. Here, we will examine some of the key preconditions for the formulation of national policy around practice integration. The reader is referred to Manderscheid (2012) for a full explanation of the process of national policy formulation (see also Box 7–1 for a brief overview of policy development).

System is the typical structure, patterns of care, and providers made available to an individual with behavioral health conditions. Until recently, behavioral care has been separated from medical care in offices and organizations with virtually no clinical linkages to primary care. Since the beginning of modern community mental health care in the 1950s and 1960s, and community substance use care in the 1970s, a clear and determined effort has been made to maintain this service separation until very recently. Some of the subsequent challenges that have arisen due to this long-term separation will be described later in this chapter (see the section "Practice Implementation and System Integration").

Subsequent sections will examine the key phases of the development of policy content, the evolution of practice, and the manner by which policy becomes practice. These concepts will then be applied to integrated care practice. Finally, some speculations will be offered about the likely future of integrated care.

Box 7-1. Policy Development: A brief overview

Formal policy development is usually intended to respond to a problem identified through research or advocacy, or both. The developmental trajectory almost always moves from a less formal statement, to a more formal statement, and to a law, although not all policy formulations actually become law. These developmental phases address the evolution of policy content rather than policy process.

In a similar manner, the process of policy development usually occurs over the course of several key steps (Manderscheid 2012). First, a credible national source becomes a champion for the policy. Subsequently, the policy is affirmed by one or more credible national groups representing a broad range of interests around the topic. Finally, key groups advocate for regulatory or legislative reform to codify the policy.

POLICY DEVELOPMENT FOR INTEGRATED CARE

Despite a common belief that integration of primary care and behavioral health is a new policy trend, in actuality the discussion began decades ago. As early as the mid-1980s, the National Institute of Mental Health and the mental health field came to recognize that the prevalence of chronic diseases, such as heart disease and diabetes, was disproportionately higher in persons with serious mental illness. The definition of a *person with serious mental illness* used here is that promulgated by the Substance Abuse and Mental Health Services Administration (SAMHSA): a person with a mental illness has serious impairment of his or her functioning in the family, at work and/or school, and in the community (U.S. Department of Health and Human Services 1999a). These chronic diseases were not only more prevalent in this population, but they also occurred at an earlier age than in the general population (McCarrick et al. 1986). As a result, consideration was given at the time to the potential of training primary care physicians to serve as case managers for adults with serious mental illness (Regier et al. 1985). However, during the late 1980s, the national government was not particularly welcoming to broad policy innovations around mental health services. Hence, these practices were not implemented into service delivery.

Early in the 1990s, considerable time and effort was spent thinking through the Health Security Act proposed during the administration of President William J. Clinton. Like the much later Patient Protection and Affordable Care Act (ACA) policy, the proposed Health Security Act would have centered the health care system in primary care. Within the Clinton framework, mental health and substance use care would have become specialties affiliated with primary care, much as cardiac care is today. Subsequently, after almost 2 years of acrimonious debate, the proposed Health Security Act was not passed by the Congress.

In 1999, then Surgeon General David Satcher published the first-ever Surgeon General's report on mental health in the 200-year history of the U.S. Public Health Service (U.S. Department of Health and Human Services 1999b). This report was notable in two respects. First, Surgeon General Satcher documented that mental health treatment works and has a sound scientific base. Second, he called for the integration of mental health and primary care during the following decade.

One year later, in 2000, Surgeon General Satcher organized a meeting on mental health–primary care integration at The Carter Center in Atlanta. This was a landmark meeting not only because it produced a second Surgeon General's report on service integration (U.S. Department of Health and Human Services 2001), but also because it outlined major tasks that would be necessary for the U.S. Department of Health and Human Services to accomplish if practice integration were to become successful. Work on those tasks, such as program coordination between SAMHSA and the Health Resources and Services Administration (HRSA), began immediately and continues to the present day.

In 2003, the administration of President George W. Bush published the report of the President's New Freedom Commission on Mental Health 2003. The very first principle elucidated in that report focused on practice integration: There can be no good health without good mental health, and vice versa. As an outcome of that report, SAMHSA commissioned a study by the Institute of Medicine on the key dimensions of service integration. The final report of that project, *Improving the Quality of Health Care for Mental and Substance-Use Conditions* (Institute of Medicine 2006), provided very practical information on how care could be integrated in clinical settings.

Also in 2006, Craig Colton and I (R.M.) published the first-ever state-level mortality data on persons with serious mental illness who were served in public mental health systems (Colton and Manderscheid 2006). The findings were both devastating and discouraging: Public mental health patients were dying 25 years prematurely, on average, in part because they lacked access to any primary care services. In large measure, these findings shaped and focused the subsequent national political debate about system and practice-level integration. Facilitated by the 2008 Paul Wellstone and Pete Domenici Mental Health Parity and Addiction Equity Act, the 2010 ACA clearly moves toward full integration within a primary care framework. This landmark legislation calls for the creation of medical homes operated by primary care providers and health homes operated by behavioral health providers that offer fully integrated services.

Thus, in just 25 years, from 1985 to 2010, the national policy clearly has evolved from strong support for separated mental health and substance use systems of care to one that supports fully integrated systems and clinical practice. This policy evolution has been facilitated by research that identified major physical health problems in persons seeking behavioral health care; by a Surgeon General who called for services integration; by the New Freedom Commission, which endorsed the Surgeon General's position; and, finally, by the ACA, which codified the change into national law.

Since 2010, this policy evolution has continued. A major example of how this policy has advanced and directly impacted models of integrated care includes the development of the SAMHSA-HRSA Center for Integrated Health Solutions (www.integration.samhsa.gov) and specific funding opportunities, such as the Primary and Behavioral Health Care Integration grants, which since 2009 have funded 187 grantees across the country to integrate primary care and behavioral health (often using reverse integration models). In addition, in the last 6 years there have been continued calls for integration from the national level (Agency for Healthcare Research and Quality [AHRQ] and Centers for Medicare and Medicaid Services [CMS]) to the local level (e.g., Federally Qualified Health Centers and community mental health centers). Across the country, states view the integration of behavioral health and traditional medical care as a key ingredient to effective statewide policy and health care practice (Bachrach et al. 2014).

CHALLENGES IN PRACTICE IMPLEMENTATION

Care delivery typically evolves in response to the diffusion of evidence-based interventions that result from both clinical and services research. Frequently, these practices are taught during graduate training to new clinicians, who then bring them to care settings where they are implemented. The entire cycle from research to scientific publication, to textbook, to classroom, to practice is exceedingly long. The New Freedom Commission on Mental Health (2003) has estimated the entire cycle to be about 17 years.

Although widely employed, it is also worthwhile to note that continuing education training is notably unsuccessful in transmitting new knowledge or changing current practice. As a consequence of these difficulties, knowledge transfer programs have been developed to encourage the adoption of new evidence-based care interventions (Backer 1991). The AHRQ is an example of a health care knowledge transfer program, and the University of Washington Advancing Integrated Mental Health Solutions (AIMS) Center (https:// aims.uw.edu) is devoted to the knowledge transfer of the evidence base for the Collaborative Care Model (CoCM).

PRACTICE IMPLEMENTATION AND SYSTEM INTEGRATION

Modern system integration represents an especially complex instance of new practice implementation. It combines a clinical practice innovation (implementation of a complex treatment team spanning behavioral health and primary care providers) with a new organizational configuration at the system level (an accountable care organization that operates a network of medical and/or health homes) with a new method of paying for care (payment bundling or integrated case rates). Other examples of policy-driven system transformation advancing integration include the CMS State Innovation Model grants, Accountable Care Collaboratives, and Coordinated Care Organizations, as well as the Delivery System Reform Incentive Payment program. Each of these models focuses on integration of systems of care and direct integration of clinical practice with an interdisciplinary team approach.

In addition to its complexity, clinical practice integration simply has not evolved from clinical research to textbook, to classroom, to the clinic setting. Integrated care has come about through the more abrupt avenue of new national policy that is also forcing considerable change at the system level, as outlined in detail in the section "Policy Development for Integrated Care" earlier in this chapter. As a result, clinical and services researchers, program managers, state policy makers, and clinicians all are scrambling to catch up with the new national policy, in an environment with few practical guides to action.

It also should be noted that because integration of clinical practice and systems of care will lead to relatively large-scale changes in organizational and financial arrangements, considerable inertia and resistance exist in the behavioral health services community and, to a lesser extent, in the primary care community. Much of this fear is misplaced; however, it remains an element of slowing policy implementation.

In the next section of this chapter, "Full Integration," the future phase of clinical practice integration is outlined and the practice-level response to the new national policy is presented. For greater discussion of the phases of integration, readers are referred to a published analysis regarding future phases of service integration (Manderscheid and Kathol 2014).

FULL INTEGRATION

Full integration refers to the availability of an ongoing, integrated treatment team and an integrated financial arrangement in which behavioral health and primary care funding are in the same pool. This arrangement can exist in either a primary care or a behavioral health setting. A fully integrated treatment team permits routine and ongoing dialogue to address both behavioral and physical comorbidities at the same time. In this arrangement, an integrated treatment plan can be developed, implemented, and assessed. This arrangement can also normalize behavioral health care and reduce stigma. The actual components or core elements of effective integration are evolving, with research defining and refining effective models for integration. As outlined in Chapter 1, "Elements of Effective Design and Implementation," the CoCM is both efficacious and effective and highlights essential elements for successful implementation.

This increasing solidification of the practice model of integration provides growing opportunities to improve the interface between policy and practice. The clinical models refine and inform minute policy changes, bringing specificity to the broad national integration policy shifts. These are areas in which national and state policy implementation are still "catching up" with the broader national policy driving integration. The most common example is challenges with financing new models of care (see Chapter 8, "Financing Integrated Care") as a result of state systems with separate and often structurally different funding streams (e.g., fee-for-service vs. carve-out or capitated) for medical and behavioral health care. As an example, state agency leadership and providers in Colorado evaluated policy and administrative rule barriers to practice integration, and they published a report on the challenges both for the state system and clinical practice and recommended actions to overcome these barriers (State of Colorado 2015). This is an important step in making the national policy actionable and meaningful at the practice level—it is literally addressing layers of policy, administrative rule, and clinical practice history to achieve a new model of care. So although national policy is quite a bit ahead, implementation requires change at many subsequent levels.

A goal of full integration includes fully integrated funding, which allows the bureaucratic complexities of paying for behavioral health care and primary care under separately organized, carve-out arrangements to be eliminated.

Further, fully integrated funding is concordant with the implementation of case (per person served) and capitation (per person covered) rates, which is a primary goal of the ACA, and a new initiative of former Health and Human Services Secretary Sylvia Burwell, as described below. Finally, under this arrangement, the assurance that needed behavioral health care will be provided can be protected by appropriate performance measures (see the appendix, "Performance and Outcome Measures for Integrated Care").

In 2015, Health and Human Services Secretary Sylvia Burwell announced a value-based purchasing initiative (see www.hhs.gov/news/press/2015pres/01/20150126a.html). This initiative encompasses system reform directed toward integrated care services, as well as the implementation of performance-adjusted case rates. Further, the Secretary set very ambitious goals for this initiative around Medicare funding. Specifically, the initiative specified that 90% of federal Medicare dollars should be managed in this way by the end of 2018. Similar plans are expected for Medicaid, but there are currently no quantitative targets for the states.

Because integrated care represents large-scale system and financial change, this new care model is often perceived as threatening to behavioral health providers and traditional medical models. Although this fear is basically unfounded, as noted above, it has dampened implementation of services integration practice. The expectation is that these fears will be mitigated as services integration becomes more common. In Appendix 7–A, Table 1 provides an outline of the phases of integration, and Table 2 provides additional information on exemplars of practice integration. A quick review will lead to several key conclusions. First, practice integration is being implemented by using a broad array of underlying organizational, financial, and clinical models. Second, these developments are taking place throughout the United States in a diverse set of political and system contexts. Third, these pilot efforts give hope, hold lessons, and provide direction for those just beginning on the journey of clinical integration.

At the same time, these new integration efforts will be inhibited by a broad range of impediments, as well as facilitated by factors that promote them. In Appendix 7–A, Table 3 summarizes several categories of key impediments and key facilitators of practice integration that focus primarily on the delivery of services. These include care delivery, education, administration and finances, practice issues, and social and/or environmental factors.

Because practice integration is a complex transformation, these impediments and facilitators also are complex. Those undertaking clinical integration efforts should review these impediments and facilitators for applicability to their own program efforts. Some impediments likely will require work-arounds; some facilitators can be employed to accelerate implementation. Awareness and vigilance in remaining informed are central to eliminating myths about barriers as well as refining where change is still needed.

Because policy and practice of integration are changing so rapidly, it is important that parties from both levels of change are aware of changes at the other level. Providers often blame state and federal regulations for slowing the practice implementation of the model. Although real challenges to integration remain, some studies have demonstrated that providers remain mired in barrier myths rather than genuine administrative or policy rule challenges (see one example of this analysis in State of Colorado [2015]). It is vital that providers remain aware of changes being made at all policy levels to address barriers and to improve integration of services. They can inform as well as take advantage of these changes.

It also is important to take a step back to examine the broader level of our institutional structures to determine how they facilitate or impede practice integration. This is demonstrated in Appendix 7–A, Table 4. The major institutional domains included in this table are organizational integration and adaptation, funding integration and adaptation, pattern maintenance, and goal attainment. Together, these are the fundamental imperatives for the survival of any system. In each domain, several inhibitors are still operative. However, also in each domain, solutions and work-arounds are available for each of these inhibitors. In Appendix 7–A, Tables 3 and 4 outline some of the challenges that remain in the translation between policy, regulation, and practice—the evolution of national policy to clinical care.

FUTURE OF INTEGRATED CARE

As we move toward the future, it is very important to take note of some facts about the present. One very important benchmark is our national health care spending. It is shocking to note that more than 27.5% or $444 billion of our national health care spending in 2012 was for persons with behavioral health conditions. It also is very important to note that only 6.8% or $91.8 billion was spent on specialty behavioral health care (Melek et al. 2012). Clearly, we can predict that good integrated care has great potential to reduce the overall total cost of care for behavioral health patients, whether they are served in health homes or medical homes. This dictum will play a huge role in the future evolution of clinical integration and adaptation in policy. Thus, with the policy backdrop described above, the practice incentives introduced by the ACA, and the financial dictum just described, clinical practice integration not only will become inevitable, it also will be implemented at an accelerating pace.

Within the next decade, we can expect integrated medical homes operated out of the primary care sector to serve up to 90% of persons with behavioral health conditions, and integrated health homes operated out of the behavioral health sector to serve about 10%. However, as a result of the implementation of the ACA, the behavioral health care service population also is likely to double in size during the next 10 years. Hence, integrated health homes operated by behavioral health care entities will then be serving about as many patients as are served by behavioral health providers today. Developments resulting from the replacement of the ACA remain to be seen as of this writing.

To conclude, in the short-term future, behavioral health care is on the cusp of major, foundational changes. As we move toward fully integrated treatment teams and fully integrated financing, much better care and better access to care will be provided for patients with mental health and substance use conditions, while behavioral health access will also improve for patients in primary care. Integrated health homes and integrated medical homes operated by these teams and with these financing structures will be able to address the chronic health problems first identified in behavioral health care patients more than 30 years ago. All of this provides good reasons to be very optimistic about the future.

REFERENCES

Agency for Healthcare Research and Quality: A Guidebook of Professional Practices for Behavioral Health and Primary Care Integration: Observations from Exemplary Sites (AHRQ Publ No 14-0070-1-EF). Rockville, MD, Agency for Healthcare Research and Quality, March 2015. Availabe at: https://integrationacademy.ahrq.gov/sites/default/files/AHRQ_AcademyGuidebook.pdf. Accessed March 2, 2017.

Bachrach D, Anthony S, Detty A: State strategies for integrating physical and behavioral health services in a changing Medicaid environment. The Commonwealth Fund, 2014. Available at: http://www.commonwealthfund.org/~/media/files/publications/fund-report/2014/aug/1767_bachrach_state_strategies_integrating_phys_behavioral_hlt_827.pdf#sthash.jAwfqkdy.dpuf. Accessed September 21, 2016.

Backer TE: Knowledge utilization: the third wave. Sci Commun 12(3):225–240, 1991

Colton CW, Manderscheid RW: Congruencies in increased mortality rates, years of potential life lost, and causes of death among public mental health clients in eight states. Prev Chronic Dis 3(2):A42, 2006 16539783

Dundon M, Dollar K, Schohn M, Lantinga LJ: Primary Care-Mental Health Integration: Co-Located, Collaborative Care: An Operations Manual. VA Center for Integrated Health Care, March 2011. Available at: http://www.mirecc.va.gov/cih-visn2/Documents/Clinical/MH-IPC_CCC_Operations_Manual_Version_2_1.pdf. Accessed March 2, 2017.

Institute of Medicine, Committee on Crossing the Quality Chasm: Adaptation to Mental Health and Addictive Disorders: Improving the Quality of Health Care for Mental and Substance-Use Conditions. Washington, DC, National Academies Press, 2006

Jolles MP, Haynes-Maslow L, Roberts MC, et al: Mental health service use for adult patients with co-occurring depression and physical chronic health care needs, 2007–2010. Med Care 53(8):708–712, 2015 26147863

Manderscheid RW: Formulation of mental health policy in the United States, with comparative case studies of South Africa and Thailand, in 21st Century Global Mental Health. Edited by Sorel ES. Burlington, MA, Jones & Bartlett Learning, 2012, pp 351–364

Manderscheid R, Kathol R: Fostering sustainable, integrated medical and behavioral health services in medical settings. Ann Intern Med 160(1):61–65, 2014 24573665

McCarrick AK, Manderscheid, RW, Bertolucci DE, et al: Chronic medical problems in the chronically mentally ill. Hosp Community Psychiatry 37(3):289–291, 1986 3957277

Melek S, Norris DT, Paulus J: Economic Impact of Integrated Medical-Behavioral Healthcare: Implications for Psychiatry. Chicago, IL, Milliman, 2012

New Freedom Commission on Mental Health: Achieving the Promise: Transforming Mental Health Care in America: Final Report (DHHS Publ No SMA-03–3832). Rockville, MD, U.S. Department of Health and Human Services, 2003

Regier DA, Burke JD Jr, Manderscheid RW, et al: The chronically mentally ill in primary care. Psychol Med 15(2):265–273, 1985 4023131

State of Colorado: Tri-Agency Regulatory Alignment Initiative to Support Integrated Care: Report. Convened by Colorado Departments of Human Services-Office of Behavioral Health, Health Care Policy and Financing, and Public Health and Environment. Office of Behavioral Health, 2015. Available at: https:// drive.google.com/file/d/0B6eUVZvBBTHjekVCRzJBN3lpZFk/ view?pref=2andpli=1. Accessed September 22, 2016.

U.S. Department of Health and Human Services: Estimation: methodology for adults with serious mental illness (SMI). Federal Register, June 24, 1999a. Available at: https://www.gpo.gov/fdsys/pkg/FR-1999-06-24/pdf/99-15377.pdf. Accessed September 22, 2016.

U.S. Department of Health and Human Services: Mental Health: A Report of the Surgeon General. Rockville, MD, U.S. Department of Health and Human Services, Substance Abuse and Mental Health Services Administration, Center for Mental Health Services, National Institutes of Health, National Institute of Mental Health, 1999b

U.S. Department of Health and Human Services: Report of a Surgeon General's Working Meeting on the Integration of Mental Health Services and Primary Health Care. Held on November 30–December 1, 2000, at The Carter Center, Atlanta, Georgia. Rockville, MD, Office of the Surgeon General, 2001

APPENDIX 7–A

Tables of Key Factors in Integrated Care: Phases, Models, Impediments, and Facilitators

TABLE 1. Phases of integration: integrated care components

Variable	Model 1 (treat-refer)	Model 2 (bidirectional)	Model 3 (full)
Access	Discrete and nonoverlapping medical and behavioral health (BH) provider groups and treatment settings; frequent delays	Non-network cross-disciplinary providers at primary service delivery site; selective access	Integrated medical and BH network providers uniformly present in service locations; ready access
Integrated care delivery	Clinician documentation of information firewalls; crisis-dictated communication and care coordination; nonexistent continuity	Site-specific cross-disciplinary information access, communication, and care coordination; partial continuity	Full integrated medical and BH network provider information access, communication, care coordination, and continuity
Payment	Separate medical and BH benefits, claims adjudication procedures, and coding and billing rules	Separate medical and BH benefits, claims adjudication procedures, and coding and billing rules; subsidized cross-disciplinary services	Consolidated medical and BH benefit set, claims adjudication procedures, and coding and billing rules

TABLE 1. Phases of integration: integrated care components *(continued)*

Variable	Model 1 (treat-refer)	Model 2 (bidirectional)	Model 3 (full)
Outcomes	Discipline-specific clinical and cost and/or savings accountability	Discipline-specific clinical and cross-disciplinary cost and/or savings accountability	Medical and BH clinical and cost and/or savings accountability

Source. Adapted from Manderscheid and Kathol 2014.

TABLE 2.   Examples of exemplary models and initiatives

Title or type	Funding organization	Model or initiative description
Advancing Care Together (ACT): A whole person approach to health care	ACT is funded by the Colorado Health Foundation and housed in the Department of Family Medicine at the University of Colorado Denver. It supports 11 practice sites with over 440 clinicians and over 120,000 patients.	The 4-year, three-phase ACT program wants to make every door the right door to care by altering practice in primary care practices and community mental health centers across settings and populations. Demonstration grants enabled disparate programs to identify, test, and evaluate promising ways to integrate care for patients in both primary care and community mental health settings. The best practices identified by the program are being shared with Colorado practices looking to integrate patient care, and with other practices nationwide.
Collaborative Care Model (CoCM)	University of Washington Advancing Integrated Mental Health Solutions (AIMS) Center	A broader application of the Improving Mood—Providing Access to Collaborative Treatment (IMPACT) program, the CoCM emphasizes collaborations among primary care providers, care managers, and psychiatric consultants to provide care and monitor patients' progress. The model has led to improved clinical outcomes and lower costs, spanning a variety of mental disorders, settings, and payment mechanisms. The program is an outgrowth of what is often called consultation-liaison psychiatry. The University of Washington AIMS Center—first established following the success of the IMPACT and DIAMOND (Depression Improvement Across Minnesota, Offering a New Direction) programs—develops, tests, and helps implement collaborative care, providing coaching and implementation support, education, and workforce development.

TABLE 2. Examples of exemplary models and initiatives *(continued)*

Title or type	Funding organization	Model or initiative description
Coordinated Care Organizations (CCOs)	State of Oregon—statewide program	Following a CMS waiver granted several years ago, Oregon established 16 regional CCOs to deliver health care and coverage for people eligible for the Oregon Health Plan (Medicaid), including individuals who are dually Medicare-Medicaid eligible. With fixed budgets, the CCOs operate patient-centered, team-led care models that emphasize one-stop care and services. They are to deliver defined outcomes based on the use of best practices and integrated services, within the fixed budget provided. The state estimates that this approach to integrated care for the Medicaid and dual eligible population can realize a potential savings of $3 billion over 5 years.
Integration Workforce Study	This project is undertaken by the Oregon Health & Science University and funded by the Agency for Healthcare Research and Quality (AHRQ), the Maine Health Access Foundation, and the California Mental Health Services Authority.	The Integration Workforce Study helped identify and assess the range of competencies and practices needed by primary care and behavioral health professionals to engage successfully in integrated care. The eight study sites across the United States were chosen based on their differing levels of duration and maturity of their integration efforts. The outcome of the study included creation of *A Guidebook of Professional Practices for Behavioral Health and Primary Care Integration: Observations from Exemplary Sites* (AHRQ 2015).

TABLE 2.   Examples of exemplary models and initiatives (*continued*)

Title or type	Funding organization	Model or initiative description
Medicaid health homes	Nationwide models, funded by the CMS and the Center for Health Care Strategies	Using ACA funds, Medicaid health homes provide states with a mechanism to support better care management for people with complex health needs, with the goal of improving health outcomes and curbing costs. As of September 2015, 19 states and Washington, DC, have 27 operating Medicaid health home models. Integrated care (behavioral and physical) is the specific focus of 6 states (AL, ID, NY, RI, SD, WA). The work in these states could inform other states considering this model.
Private sector integrated care model	Intermountain Healthcare, Salt Lake City, UT, is a nonprofit confederation of 22 hospitals and over 185 clinics across the state.	Over the course of several decades, Intermountain has developed and grown a program that integrates behavioral health professionals in the primary care setting while also folding in community resources, care management, and patient-family engagement. Patients with depression treated in these integration clinics are 54% less likely to visit emergency departments. In addition, patients treated in the integrated clinics have a 27% lower rate of cost growth. The success of this program has resulted in its replication in ME, MI, NH, OR, and local UT state agencies.

TABLE 2. Examples of exemplary models and initiatives *(continued)*

Title or type	Funding organization	Mode or initiative description
Sustaining Healthcare Across Integrated Primary Care Efforts (SHAPE)	Colorado-based Rocky Mountain Health Plans, the Department of Family Medicine at the University of Colorado Denver, and the Collaborative Family Healthcare Association of Colorado; part of the Medicaid Prime project (see section "Rocky Mountain Health Plans" in Chapter 8, "Financing Integrated Care")	The SHAPE program, established in 2012 as a pilot program, has been comparing three western Colorado practices with integrated behavioral health and global payments to pay for team-based care, with a control group of three integrated practices using fee-for-service payments. The program's aim is both to make behavioral health providers part of the primary care team and to move away from fee-for-service-based practice. Participating practices can lose payments if they don't meet quality and cost targets; they can get incentives for improved health outcomes. In 18 months, there was a 5.5% reduction in Medicaid spending across the three global payment practices.
TEAMcare model	University of Washington AIMS Center and Group Health Research Institute, funded by the National Institute of Mental Health	The TEAMcare approach—consistent with earlier studies that emphasized "consultation-liaison psychiatry"—encourages simultaneous treatment of all conditions experienced by individuals with comorbid mental and physical health problems, such as depression that co-occurs with diabetes or cardiovascular disease. The model is modeled on IMPACT and is designed to prevent situations in which one poorly controlled chronic condition lessens the effectiveness of the treatment of another.

TABLE 2.   Examples of exemplary models and initiatives *(continued)*

Title or type	Funding organization	Model or initiative description
Veterans' Primary Care-Mental Health Integration	U.S. Department of Veterans Affairs (VA), Veterans Health Administration	The VA—through its Veterans Health Administration—has pioneered clinical programs of integrated care for those it serves for many years, recognizing that body and mind are both involved in healing. The identification of posttraumatic stress disorder as a comorbid illness alongside physical ailments in veterans helped move programs and policy toward a more integrated approach. Indeed, the VA developed and disseminated its operations manual on primary care–mental health integration programs with co-located, collaborative care to promote integrated care first in 2005, and has updated and recirculated the manual as recently as 2011 (see Dundon et al. 2011). The manual continues to serve as a prototype not only for integrated care at VA Medical Center facilities but for integrated care at public and private sector facilities nationwide.

TABLE 2. Examples of exemplary models and initiatives *(continued)*

Title or type	Funding organization	Model or initiative description
Virginia Integrated Care Initiative	The Virginia Association of Community Service Boards received funds from the Virginia Health Care Foundation to test local models of integrated care.	The Virginia Integrated Care Initiative arose as early as 2012 following failed efforts to bring about enacted legislation to advance integrated care programs under the state's Medicaid program. The program—with funds being made available to local CSBs (all behavioral health entities)—are establishing and testing models that bring primary care services to people receiving services in CSBs around the state (e.g., Arlington, Loudoun, and Fairfax County CSBs in Northern Virginia; Norfolk, Hampton, and Chesapeake CSBs in the Tidewater area). Based on outcomes, the models will be grown throughout the Virginia CSBs statewide.

Note.   ACA=Affordable Care Act; CMS=Centers for Medicare and Medicaid Services; CSB=community service board.

TABLE 3. Integration impediments and facilitators

Impediments	Facilitators
Care delivery	
Insurance prohibitions denying two or more medical encounters in the same day (this has been resolved in numerous states but remains a commonly misunderstood concern for providers).	CMS's ACA Section 2703 Health Home Program, promoting integrated care.
Overly restrictive managed care practices for behavioral health care.	Reduction of coverage breaks by state Medicaid 1115 waivers limiting the number of times a person's eligibility is scrutinized in a given year.
Use of insurance preapproval requirements to thwart side-by-side work by behavioral health care and primary care providers.	Improved interoperability across facilities and practices, facilitating shared use of medical records among collaborating clinicians.
Patient privacy laws and regulations that prevent providers from sharing information about mental, substance use, and physical disorders (42 Code of Federal Regulations Part II is often cited as a concern).	SAMHSA-HRSA Center for Integrated Health Solutions, including models of integrated care and technical assistance to entities seeking to create integrated systems.
Practice of Medicaid and private insurers to disenroll from insurance rather than suspend coverage when people become incarcerated.	States that suspend, not disenroll, people from health insurance coverage when entering the corrections system, enabling easier coverage reinstatement after adjudication and following release.

TABLE 3. Integration impediments and facilitators *(continued)*

Impediments	Facilitators
	Education
Inadequate clinical training about the practice and benefits of integrated care.	Yale University School of Medicine has established a new Department of Psychiatry program: the Psychological Medicine Service designed to prepare medical clinicians across disciplines and other health care professionals for a health care system moving toward multidisciplinary integrated care.
Siloed education systems that separate training in physical and behavioral health care.	
Insufficient cross-professional team training for collaborating service providers.	American Psychiatric Association Support and Alignment grant to train 3,500 psychiatrists in the CoCM and the University of Washington's model curriculum for integrated care for psychiatry residents.
	SAMHSA–HRSA Center for Integrated Health Solutions, including core education and both training competencies and national training resources for high-quality integrated care.
	University of Michigan's School of Social Work program focused on an integrated model of care.

TABLE 3.   Integration impediments and facilitators *(continued)*

Impediments	Facilitators
Administration and finances	
Financing silos that separate physical and behavioral health care research, education, services, and service coverage from each other.	States, counties, and care organizations that merge separate agencies and offices for physical and behavioral health care to foster integration.
Fear of losing research, education, services, and brick-and-mortar funding streams as the result of policies that would end silos and integrate funding as well as care.	Greater focus on private and public foundation resources that historically support integrated care, coupled with a growing number of federal dollars enabling communities to pilot best practice, integrated care programs.
Funders' use of separate provider networks, billing and coding practices, and record-keeping requirements for physical and behavioral care.	CMS's ACA Section 2703 Health Home Program giving states a new tool to develop more person-centered models of coordinated care that potentially reduce costs for this high-need population.
	Improved service provider record interoperability (e.g., new Los Angeles County initiative enabling behavioral health and primary care clinicians to safely and securely share vital, patient-authorized data in real time—often at co-located facilities—to treat the mind and body).

TABLE 3. Integration impediments and facilitators *(continued)*

Impediments	Facilitators
Practice issues	
Difficulty determining which provider organization—behavioral health or primary care—will lead an integrated care program.	Growing number of evidence-based best practices and models of integrated care that can serve different populations, ages, and communities.
Inadequate and/or insufficient day-to-day collaboration among members of a cross-professional integrated care team.	Technical assistance available from CMS's Health Home Information Resource Center to help state Medicaid agencies—and localities—develop and implement health home models meeting unique goals and needs.
Indecision regarding the identification of the best integrated care model to adopt in a particular location for a particular population.	The U.S. Department of Veterans Affairs revised operations manual, *Primary Care–Mental Health Integration: Co-Located, Collaborative Care* (Dundon et al. 2011), is a how-to about creating successful and sustainable co-located, collaborative care primary care–mental health integration programs.
Interpersonal conflict over team leadership for individual patient care.	In partnership with the New York State Department of Health, and with support from the New York State Health Foundation, the Center for Health Care Strategies created a Health Homes Learning Collaborative to identify and share best practices in health home design and implementation.

TABLE 3.   Integration impediments and facilitators *(continued)*

Impediments	Facilitators
	Practice issues *(continued)*
	The Yale University Department of Psychiatry's Connecticut Mental Health Center, a medical home to 600 or more behavioral health patients, partners with Cornell Scott-Hill Health Center to provide all the benefits of primary care at the mental health center in a "reverse" health home.
Social and/or environmental factors	
Stigma related to behavioral health as a repellent that keeps programs, policies, and practices from coming together as integrated care (e.g., fear of shared waiting rooms).	Anti-stigma campaigns to educate the public and health care staff about mental health issues, how to best communicate with people with behavioral problems, and how to avoid stigmatizing behaviors. (For example, a new program just initiated in New York City, ThriveNYC, is designed to help "change the culture" about mental health.)
Insufficiently trained front-desk and other staff regarding proper ways to engage patients (e.g., inadvertent "labeling," insufficient attention to confidentiality issues).	Training and education programs, such as Mental Health First Aid, train providers, schools, clergy, first responders, and laypeople how to respond when someone has a panic attack, psychotic episode, or appears depressed or suicidal.

Note.   ACA = Affordable Care Act; CMS = Centers for medicare and Medicaid Services; SAMHSA-HRSA = Substance Abuse and Mental Health Services Administration–Health Resources and Services Administration.

TABLE 4.   Institutional inhibitors and facilitators of integrated care elements

Focal issue	Selected inhibitor	Selected facilitator
Integration and adaptation: organizational	Government agencies and offices are structured and function within individual care areas (e.g., separate agencies for physical and behavioral illness services and programs; separate agencies and offices for research on specific disease categories).	The structure of regulations and administrative functions can simplify and improve program coordination and facilitate access, eligibility, and resource management. They can be accomplished through such means as the following:
	Treatment sites and health care professionals often are segregated by disease entity.	• Coordinating programs and grants across agencies and offices.
		• Reorganizing offices and agencies and treatment sites across care areas (e.g., SAMHSA-HRSA Center for Integrated Health Solutions and cross-specialty training programs; CMS integrated care initiative and resources).
		• Considering and implementing joint management at all levels, from federal programs and grant mechanisms through community-based health care service.

TABLE 4. Institutional inhibitors and facilitators of integrated care elements *(continued)*

Focal issue	Selected inhibitor	Selected facilitator
Integration and adaptation: funding	The division, structure, and flow of funds for health and social care and related services can affect virtually all aspects of integrated care. • Funding for health care services, supportive services, and research generally is separated and restricted by disorder. • Insurance coverage—whether public or private—is focused on separate illnesses and individual encounters with the treatment system. • Covered diagnosis and medical necessity are requirements for individuals to receive any behavioral health services. • Some services may not be covered by insurance when separate treatment for co-occurring disorders takes place on the same day. • Billing may be linked to treatment site, precluding payment for behavioral health care coverage in primary care settings.	Broaden programs such as CMS Accountable Health Communities model, extending federal Medicaid financial participation to mechanisms that enable health care entities to identify and address patients' supportive services needs. Expand ACA program and funding related to integrated care. Eliminate public and private sector impediments to reimbursement for same-day services for the treatment of multiple disorders in a single person. Encourage pooled funds across programs, agencies, or departments in both grant making and program development to promote integrated care across disciplines to focus on the whole person.

TABLE 4. Institutional inhibitors and facilitators of integrated care elements *(continued)*

Focal issue	Selected inhibitor	Selected facilitator
Pattern maintenance	The mode of service delivery and management—how staff are trained, perform their responsibilities and tasks, work together, and relate to patients and family caregivers and their needs—has a major impact on a number of critical variables in integrated care. • Health care professional training occurs primarily by body function, patient age group, disease entity, and professional interest. Specialty training most often occurs in physically separate sites, without consideration of the prevention, diagnosis, or management of comorbid conditions. • Treatment sites segregate behavioral health patients from other patients.	• Restructure health care professional training to emphasize the relationship between behavioral and physical health, their interactions, and the importance of a whole person approach to care, consistent with the new integrated models of care being implemented around the country. Physically integrate behavioral and physical health care education in both didactic and hands-on aspects of health care education. • Co-locate service programs, whether within behavioral health or primary care settings, and establish programs of integrated records as well as comprehensive team-based diagnosis, treatment, and follow-up care and planning. • Address privacy rules and policy to support shared documentation, shared treatment, and reduction of stigma on specific conditions.

TABLE 4.   Institutional inhibitors and facilitators of integrated care elements *(continued)*

Focal issue	Selected inhibitor	Selected facilitator
Pattern maintenance *(continued)*	• Privacy laws require segregated behavioral health and physical health records. • Behavioral health treatment plans must be managed separately from physical health treatment plans because of disparate regulatory and insurance requirements.	• Adopt the concept of health homes that link behavioral and physical care in an integrated fashion to change the current pattern emphasizing segregated care systems. • Reduce regulatory requirements for behavioral health documentation; particularly for services offered in medical settings.
Goal attainment	Measurement of success is gauged most often by counting episodes of successful prevention of or recovery from specific disease states. Federal requirements for submission of specific data on behavioral health services are separate from physical health services.	Outcome measures should be based on overall health status, not merely aggregated data related to prevention or treatment of separate disease states. Existing best practices in integrated care (see Table 2) have been subject to evaluation studies; these evaluation and measurement results should be explored as potential tools for larger assessments of integrated care results.

Note.   ACA = Affordable Care Act; CMS = Centers for medicare and Medicaid Services; SAMHSA-HRSA = Substance Abuse and Mental Health Services Administration–Health Resources and Services Administration.

CHAPTER 8

Financing Integrated Care

Kristan McIntosh, L.M.S.W.

Gaylee Morgan, M.P.P.

Rob Werner, B.A.

The evidence of the clinical and economic benefits of integrated care is extensive and compelling, but far less clear are concrete answers to the question of how to pay for it. This chapter will review the major reasons why, despite proven benefits, many organizations providing integrated care continue to struggle with sustainable financing models.

BACKGROUND AND BARRIERS TO INTEGRATED CARE

A large and growing body of research demonstrates the economic justification for integrating primary care and behavioral health, but much of it describes savings at the macro societal level, rather than quantifying savings that might be achievable at the organizational or programmatic level. In 2012, the additional health care costs incurred by people with behavioral comorbidities were estimated to be $293 billion across commercially insured, Medicaid, and Medicare beneficiaries in the United States, and through the use of effective integrated care, an estimated 9%–16% of this total amount (equating to $26–$48 billion) can be saved across the system (Melek et al. 2014). A study of the Georgia Medicaid population revealed the cost of providing mental health treatment was entirely paid for by the medical cost savings of $1,500 per patient over 2 years (California Primary Care Association 2007). Further, a meta-analysis of 57 controlled studies of the cost savings for integrated care models demonstrates an average cost savings of 27% (Mountainview Consulting Group 2016).

Another significant body of research focuses on the economic benefits of integrated care for specific conditions or populations, with much of the research focused on individuals with co-occurring diagnoses of depression and chronic medical conditions. Rafeyan (2012) found that in populations with a high burden of alcoholism or depression, integration adds $264 in costs of care per individual. However, an individual's treatment success rate and overall patient adherence to treatment doubles with this expenditure, resulting in a savings of $491 per individual treated. A large study examining the effects of the Improving Mood—Promoting Access to Collaborative Treatment (IMPACT) study for individuals with diabetes and depression found that individuals who received IMPACT experienced 115 more depression-free days over 24 months than those in the usual treatment group, which resulted in net cost-of-care savings of $1,129 over that same time period (Katon et al. 2006). In a longitudinal randomized controlled trial of IMPACT with older depressed patients (Unützer et al. 2008), results indicated that IMPACT patients had lower mean total health care costs ($29,422 vs. $32,785) over a 4-year period, a return on investment of $6 for every $1 spent for the collaborative care intervention. The study suggested an 87% probability that the IMPACT model was associated with lower health care costs when compared to usual care.

Although the research on the cost-effectiveness and long-term return on investment of health care integration is only in its infancy, it is clear that integration results in improved care and savings for the system at large. In addition, integrated care is increasingly being recognized as the preferred infrastructure for the delivery of health systems across the nation, especially with the evolution of the patient-centered medical home and accountable care organizations (ACOs) over the past 10 years (Colorado Health Foundation 2012). However, the question still remains: Why do health systems and individual practices continue to be so challenged to sufficiently cover their costs for providing integrated primary care and behavioral health services? The easy answer is that there is a classic mismatch between the two sides of the ledger: costs and revenues. Integrated care requires organizations to take on costs and provide services that are often not reimbursed under traditional fee-for-service payment models. The more fundamental answer to this question, however, is a bit more complicated and lies in the misalignment of incentives that underscore fee-for-service reimbursement models.

Onetime and Ongoing Costs

The financial efficiencies that stem from the implementation of integrated care models are concentrated in longer term cost savings. In the short term, start-up and infrastructure development costs, such as reconfiguring physical work space and information technology, are likely to be significant, and many entities are required to absorb these costs at the outset with an eye to the long-term gains (Klein and Hostetter 2014). In addition, the provision of integrated care incurs substantial costs beyond clinician time with the patient that is oftentimes unfunded through traditional payment mechanisms, including ongoing personnel (re)training, registry management and caseload review, curbside and warm handoff consultations, outreach to patients who are not engaging, and sometimes the provision of care by nonlicensed staff. Many entities that received Primary and Behavioral Health Care Integration grants from the Substance Abuse and Mental Health Services Administration (SAMHSA) have cited difficulties sustaining wellness and care management services in particular beyond the grant funding period, as these services are generally not billable under traditional models (SAMHSA-HRSA Center for Integrated Health Solutions 2014). Several organizations currently engaged in the implementation of integrated care cite numerous examples of "unfunded" organizational costs that were critical for the success of their program, including the following:

- Health information technology costs in establishing an interface between behavioral and physical health records systems (or purchasing a single system) or developing reporting capabilities to support integrated care
- Training costs including, but not limited to, educating clinical and nonclinical staff on team-based care practices and sensitivity to behavioral health conditions
- Staff positions, such as patient navigators, who are typically not billable
- Support for operational and organizational changes that are central to successful clinical integration (e.g., changes in billing, credentialing, and data reporting), all of which take additional administrative staff time

Boston Medical Center is covering the cost of adding social workers, psychiatric nurse practitioners, and patient navigators into its family medicine practices on a trial basis. Part of the rationale is that the investment may help the medical center succeed in future value-based contracts or as an ACO, by allowing it to share in any savings that accrue from improving outcomes and reducing costs.

In addition to organizational costs, in a fee-for-service environment there are nonbillable clinical services, such as the following:

- Warm handoffs between the primary care provider (PCP) and behavioral health provider (BHP), and therapeutic interventions too short to meet the requirements for a diagnostic assessment or therapy session
- "Indirect" services such as curbside consultations between the psychiatric consultant and BHP or PCP
- Time to enter data into the registry and analyze the data to identify patients who are not improving as expected, have not engaged, or have fallen out of treatment
- Time (approximately an hour a week) for the caseload-based registry review between the BHP and the psychiatric consultant
- Weekly to monthly interdisciplinary complex care meetings to discuss patient treatment strategies

In addition to these costs, which are concrete and quantifiable, organizations also report more difficult-to-quantify costs related to clinical and operational inefficiencies and challenges. These costs include the time it takes an organization to engage a true culture shift in the philosophy and clinical practice of care (see Chapter 2, "Organizational Leadership and Culture Change," and Chapter 3, "Team Development and Culture"); the time required to ensure that nonbillable huddles and staff meetings (integral to coordination among providers) are effective, efficient, and institutionalized; information technology challenges resulting from attempts to "bridge" the behavioral and physical health electronic systems (often requiring double entry); and challenges related to differences in payer contracting, credentialing, and billing across primary care and behavioral health. Compounding these challenges is that many organizations embedding integrated care models into their current practices, particularly small and medium-sized organizations and safety net organizations, lack the resources and infrastructure to quickly recognize and overcome these issues.

Reimbursement-Related Policy Barriers

Policy barriers, often relics of a fee-for-service world, have also proved to be significant obstacles to the development of sustainable financing models for integrated care (see Chapter 7, "Policy and Regulatory Environment"). For example, a number of states still do not pay for combinations of behavioral health and primary care services provided on the same day, a substantial barrier to core tenets and evidence for integration. Although much improvement has occurred in changing these policies in many localities over the past few years (Nardone et al. 2014), it remains a considerable (almost a nonstarter) barrier for some states and organizations. Other finance policy barriers that have impeded sustainable financing of these models include the following:

- Scope of practice and other restrictions that prevent certain types of licensed and nonlicensed providers from billing for services
- Telemedicine restrictions that make it difficult or, in some cases, impossible to implement this cost-effective tool to integrate care
- Place of service restrictions that limit the ability of some providers to bill for services outside the four walls of their clinic
- Carve-out policies that separate the management and payment of behavioral health and physical health services under some state Medicaid programs, making integration of care at the program level much more difficult to finance
- Medicaid managed care program design issues, including segmenting the market between large numbers of plans, creating significant administrative burden for providers, and models that do not adequately incentivize plans to develop value-based payment models

Despite these challenges, several states have taken a deliberate approach to systematically identifying and addressing policy barriers to the financing of integration in order to promote sustainability. For example, in 2011 Colorado passed legislation that directed the state's Medicaid agency to review its own policy barriers and propose solutions to promote integrated care. At the same time, the Colorado Health Foundation and the Collaborative Family Healthcare Association launched Promoting Integrated Care Sustainability, a statewide project to identify financial barriers to implementation and propose local solutions to move the model into mainstream health care (Colorado Health Foundation 2012). These and related statewide efforts have contributed to Colorado's reputation as a national leader in integration. Although policy barriers still remain for Colorado providers (e.g., behavioral health carve-out), it is clear that the state is moving toward a system that fosters sustainable integrated care.

Misaligned Incentives

In many respects, the cost and policy barriers described above are a symptom of a more fundamental barrier to integrated care: a fee-for-service reimbursement model that fails to recognize and compensate the parts of the delivery system that arguably provide the greatest value (i.e., coordination of care, wellness, and prevention services). Indeed, under a fee-for-service model, any value created by avoiding costly emergency department visits, inpatient stays, 30-day readmissions, or psychiatric institutionalization through effective integrated care accrues almost entirely to the payer. Within these systems, volume, not value, is the dominant if not the only factor driving financial decisions, including whether to invest in more effective models of care. Pay-for-performance (P4P), while a step in the right direction, is still based on a fee-for-service model, and, depending on the metrics that drive the P4P-based payment, does not necessarily reward those activities that provide the greatest value.

FINANCING MECHANISMS

Because of the barriers described above, most organizations are using a combination of approaches to finance their models. On the cost side, they are creating lean cost structures and leveraging existing resources. On the revenue side, many entities logically attempt to maximize their revenue, such as using billable staff and effectively managing the revenue cycle to ensure that billable services are consistently documented and reimbursed. Many entities discussed in this chapter also relied heavily on grant funds for start-up costs (e.g., SAMHSA Primary and Behavioral Health Care Integration grants, Health Resources and Services Administration [HRSA] Mental Health Service Expansion—Behavioral Health Integration grants, and foundation funding), and some are still reliant on these grant funds to support ongoing operations. Some organizations have developed creative approaches or workarounds to address the barriers to fiscal sustainability. These diverse strategies to sustain integrated care models are described in more detail in the next section.

Cost-Saving Strategies

Given the limitations on the revenue side of the equation (see the section "Revenue Strategies" later in this chapter), many organizations have, by necessity, taken a hard look at their expenses and experimented with creative solutions for minimizing their costs. These include leveraging existing resources and adopting innovative approaches to care.

Leveraging Existing Resources

Organizations that have or are in the process of implementing integrated care models describe conscientious efforts to leverage existing resources to the greatest extent possible. This is especially important during the start-up and initial stages of implementation. For example, the clinical leadership of the family medicine clinic at Boston Medical Center (BMC) described how they leveraged both internal and external resources to get their model off the ground with minimal expense. BMC Department of Family Medicine staff worked closely with Department of Psychiatry providers, who helped to train the agency's PCPs in the management of anxiety disorders to build PCPs' capacity to do first- and second-line evidence-based treatment. They negotiated shared clinical time for psychiatry providers across multiple BMC departments, so that they could attract and retain providers but only pay for what they needed. Leveraging their expertise to provide curbside consultation, and ultimately reduce referrals to specialty behavioral health, provided the space for the indirect approach to occur for more primary care clinics in need of consultation. They also tapped into local external groups who could train their team on strategies such as motivational interviewing and other brief interventions to enhance staff familiarity with these models.

Although BMC is a large integrated health system, some small and me-dium-sized providers have taken similar approaches to minimizing costs. Detroit Central City, a community mental health center that recently inte-grated primary care services into their clinics under a Federally Qualified Health Center (FQHC) model, cross-trained existing case management staff to also provide other enabling services. This innovation allowed them to more easily integrate services at a much lower cost than hiring new staff. Other agencies report using tiered staffing models through which they de-lineate staff functions within the integrated setting based on ability to bill (i.e., nonlicensed paraprofessional staff are responsible for wellness activities and health promotion activities, whereas licensed clinicians are nearly uni-versally focused on engaging in clinical services that are billable, such as care management) (Harris 2013).

Innovative Approaches to Care

There are also numerous examples of providers employing innovative ap-proaches to care that reduce their overall cost structure without compro-mising quality of services (Box 8–1). For example, although telemedicine can require a significant up-front investment in the necessary technology and staff training around its use, some rural providers have found it to be a highly cost-efficient investment for integrating psychiatry into their prac-tices. In New Mexico, Project ECHO (Extension for Community Healthcare Outcomes) engaged family nurse practitioners and community health work-ers in community health centers by providing additional training and sup-port to deliver behavioral health treatment, an approach that could improve cost efficiency as well as access (University of New Mexico 2015).

**Box 8–1.   Use of Certified Medical Assistants in the
DIAMOND Program**

The Entira Family Clinics, a participant in Minnesota's DIAMOND
(Depression Improvement Across Minnesota, Offering a New Direction) initiative, chose to use certified medical assistants, rather
than registered nurses or licensed therapists, as the care managers
for their depression care model. They discovered that an important
strength a care manager in their depression program must have
was patient engagement skills, so with the right manualized training and structured guidelines, certified medical assistants were
just as effective in their work with clients and significantly more
cost-effective for the program overall (Pietruszewski 2010).

Revenue Strategies

In addition to reducing costs when developing integrated care models, it is
equally important that agencies work to maximize their revenue, both during start-up to fund initial infrastructure development costs and during ongoing operations to sustain the program. Strategies to accomplish this
include obtaining government and philanthropic grants, maximizing billing, and accessing cost-based reimbursement under an FQHC model. In addition, accountable and value-based payment models can be designed to
support integrated care models, and single-payer health systems, similarly,
can create incentives that align reimbursement with integration.

Government and Philanthropic Grants

Although relying on grants to support integrated care has its risks and limitations, grant funding remains a critical component of integrated care financing. Throughout the country, there are examples of foundations and
other funders with a substantive commitment to supporting integrated care.
For example, the Sunflower Foundation in Kansas has supported education,
technical assistance, readiness assessment, transition expenses, and learning collaboratives for providers and clinicians interested in developing an integrated system (Sunflower Foundation 2015). The Social Innovation Fund
of the John A. Hartford Foundation is supporting the implementation of the
Collaborative Care Model (CoCM) at five nonprofit community health clinics throughout the Pacific Northwest (University of Washington AIMS Center 2015). And many providers have relied on grants from SAMHSA and/or
HRSA to help finance onetime costs or, in some cases, ongoing operations.

Maximize Billing

Another important strategy to sustain an integrated care program is to maximize the program's billable time. In addition to using lower-cost employees, Entira Family Clinics worked hard to ensure that their care managers were as efficient as possible and provided retraining and skills development to help them effectively increase their caseload and ability to bill for services when they could.

The codes available for billing integrated care services vary widely by state. For example, New Mexico Medicaid pays for some peer support services and whole health and wellness coaching, whereas New York Medicaid reimburses Health and Behavior codes that relate to the behavioral health components of physical conditions (e.g., smoking cessation therapy for patients with chronic obstructive pulmonary disease), and Wyoming Medicaid pays for telehealth reimbursements for psychiatric evaluations and behavioral health therapy services (Houy and Bailit 2015). The SAMHSA-HRSA Center for Integrated Health Solutions maintains current state-specific billing worksheets for all 50 states on their Web site (www.integration.samhsa.gov/financing/billing-tools#Billing). The site identifies current procedural terminology (CPT) codes that can be used to bill for integrated services.

Central to maximizing billing is investment in examining the billing and reimbursement matrix for any clinic. Organizations need to know the average reimbursement per visit and explore whether workflow or appointment adherence impacts that average. Virna Little, a national expert on billing and reimbursement for the CoCM and other models, recommends that clinics develop a grid that examines payers, staffing models, and workflow (see Appendix 8–A for an example of the grid). Each clinic needs to customize this investigation to incorporate payer information, contracts, state coding capacity, and staffing requirements for coding as well as consider workflow and efficiency. The reimbursement analysis informs the workflow and vice versa. This kind of granular assessment is an important step for organizations as they build integrated care models, and it is one of the components that takes added operational and organizational resource investment.

Cost-Based Reimbursement Under an FQHC Model

The cost-based prospective payment system (PPS), under which FQHCs are reimbursed, recognizes and compensates for some traditionally nonreimbursable costs by building them into the cost-based rate. However, some costs often remain uncompensated even with the PPS because of factors such as cost ceilings and other limitations put in place by states (i.e., how states set their thresholds for allowing providers to re-base their rate based on a change in services). In addition, while currently protected by federal law, several states have active efforts underway to try to move FQHCs toward value-based payment models. For example, California's Alternative Payment Methodology is transitioning the state away from the PPS to a payment methodology that provides the flexibility and incentives for FQHCs to deliver value over volume (California Primary Care Association 2014). Other states, including Washington (Washington State Health Care Authority 2016), Oregon (Hostetler et al. 2014), Massachusetts (Waldman et al. 2015), and New York (New York State Department of Health 2015), are currently in the early stages of similar initiatives.

Single-Payer and Vertically Integrated Health Systems

Although sometimes fodder for embattled political debates, integrated care is, in some cases, paid for by single-payer health systems for specific populations. A *single-payer system* refers to a system in which one entity (often the government) pays for care for a specific group of people, including both health and behavioral health (Rovner 2016). The U.S. Department of Defense operates such a system, called TRICARE, for active duty military and retirees, as does the U.S. Department of Veterans Affairs (VA) health care system. Through this single-payer model, the VA offers one of the most advanced programs of integrated care, called Primary Care-Mental Health Integration. Many states have explored single-payer options and have determined that single-payer systems can result in universal health care coverage and cost savings (Physicians for a National Health Program 2016), but at the time of this chapter's development, no state has moved forward with implementation.

A *vertically integrated health system* is another type of system that offers institutionalized integration as a core function of primary care (e.g., Kaiser Permanente). A vertically integrated system involves an accountable partnership among entities that provide different levels of care, such as a payer, an array of providers like physicians, academic medical centers, and long-term care facilities. These types of delivery systems can more fully benefit from the cost-effectiveness of integration because the entity is both the payer and the provider.

In both of these examples of closed systems, cost savings can be recouped when prevention and early intervention efforts (like integration) ultimately save long-term and acute costs across a population.

Accountable and Value-Based Payment Models

Large trends stemming from the Affordable Care Act (ACA), such as the Medicare Modernization Act, are pushing payer systems away from fee-for-service and toward incentive-based rewards that improve outcomes and cost efficiency (Gracey 2015). Despite several payment methodologies included in value-based payment, the general concept is the same—specific outcomes and accountability to those outcomes (value) is the metric for payment. In many cases, the value to the provider is increased as accountability is increased (for a primer on value-based payment models, variation in risk sharing, and flow of money, see Gracey 2015). Integrated care aligns with the principles of value-based payment models, which move away from the volume-based payments of fee-for-service toward payment that is tied to outcomes, thereby promoting quality and value of health care services (Brown and Crapo 2014). Managed care organizations and other payers are showing a growing interest in payment models that recognize the value of integrated care on the total cost of care. Additionally, structural changes spurred by the ACA, such as creation of Medicare and Medicaid ACOs, have furthered the idea of entities having financial responsibility for their patients (focusing systems on paying for value and cost-effective interventions). Other federal investments in health system transformation support transitions to integrated care and range from the provider level (e.g., through the Transforming Clinical Practice Initiative) all the way to the state level, through State Innovation Model planning and implementation grants. Within the Medicaid program, several states are also engaged in transformation, including value-based payment through Delivery System Reform Incentive Payment programs. Beyond federal programs, many employers and private health plans have also embraced the shift to value-based payment models.

Current funding approaches to integrated care fall along a continuum of sustainable financing. In some instances, policy barriers and antiquated payment methodologies have greatly limited the ability of providers to grow their programs. In other cases, organizations have taken a "leap of faith" that the value of integrated care will, over time, be recognized by their payers, but that the benefits for their patients warrant not waiting. At the far end of the continuum are fully (vertically and horizontally) integrated delivery systems, such as Intermountain Healthcare or Geisinger Health. These systems have been able to pioneer effective integration programs, but have had the benefit of capturing cost savings within the larger system to justify the financial commitment required for integrated behavioral health. In other words, the vertical integration between the plan and the provider components means that the incentives for integrated care are inherently aligned.

PAYMENT CASE STUDIES

As integrated health systems discover the cost benefit of integrated care for their patient populations, and as the industry moves away from a traditional fee-for-service model and toward value-based payment, support for integrated care is increasing. There are numerous examples of payers, policy makers, and providers beginning to work together to develop better and aligned payment models incorporating integrated care. These payment pilots for integration are promising, with emerging evidence of cost-effectiveness.

The DIAMOND Program: Sustaining Integrated Care

The DIAMOND program is one of the most important replications of CoCM and has been a national example of clinical success and cost-effectiveness. Initiated in 2008 by the Institute for Clinical Systems Improvement, the DIAMOND program is based on the IMPACT model of care (the foundation for the CoCM model) and incorporates universal depression screening, tracking, and monitoring (using the Patient Health Questionnaire–9) for patients in a primary care setting. The model engages a stepped care approach for treatment modification via a care team that consists of a BHP, PCP, and a psychiatric consultant. Critical to the DIAMOND program's initial financial success was the involvement of a number of health plans on the DIAMOND Steering Committee. Throughout the DIAMOND model's development and implementation, health plan representatives worked alongside providers on the steering committee. Ultimately, based on the value proposition that resulted from these steering committee conversations, the health plans created a specialized transaction code through which certified DIAMOND sites received per member per month (PMPM) reimbursement that covered depression care management, psychiatric consultation, and knowledge dissemination for up to 1 year (Institute for Clinical Systems Improvement 2014).

Today, most of the DIAMOND processes and services have been folded into Minnesota's Health Care Homes (HCH) initiative. By the time HCH certification began in 2011, DIAMOND clinics already had experience delivering integrated care, making implementation of HCH requirements (i.e., team-based care and integration of behavioral health) easier. However, because the DIAMOND model only focused on those living with major depression, additional staff training and investments were necessary to address other co-occurring behavioral health conditions within the clinics (e.g., bipolar disorder and schizophrenia). Minnesota reimburses HCH care coordination through a tiered PMPM structure, which stratifies the population and increases payment based on patient complexity. Providers who serve individuals with diagnoses of serious mental illnesses receive a small increase in the PMPM rate. However, even with this rate increase, financing the extent of care management time and activities necessary to improve outcomes for individuals with serious mental illnesses is difficult, and there is still no reimbursement of consulting psychiatric time. Therefore, several entities who participated in DIAMOND, including Entira Family Clinics, are collaborating to form ACOs that build off of their DIAMOND program models and lessons learned.

"The hope in building this ACO infrastructure is that by becoming more efficient and targeting services effectively, we will be able to show improved outcomes and cost savings. Data from the ACO is helpful [in developing a clear value proposition], and it helps push us into shared savings arrangements that we can leverage for sustainability [of our integrated care model]."—*Tim Hernandez, M.D., Entira Family Clinics*

The Mental Health Integration Program: Washington State

The Mental Health Integration Program (MHIP) has been an evolution of programming and payment reform with partnership between the state of Washington, the Community Health Plan of Washington (CHPW; a nonprofit managed care plan), and the University of Washington Advancing Integrated Mental Health Solutions (AIMS) Center. In 2004, CHPW enrolled Medicaid members from the General Assistance–Unemployable program, which was a solely state-funded program for adults deemed disabled and unable to gain employment because of a physical or mental health condition (Association for Community Affiliated Plans 2014; SAMHSA-HRSA Center for Integrated Health Solutions 2014). At the beginning of the CHPW program, the state covered medical services but not behavioral health services. The barriers to effective care became apparent, with many individuals needing care for co-occurring medical and behavioral health conditions. In 2007, CHPW, the community health clinics (CHCs), and the AIMS Center developed the MHIP model, and the state funded a pilot project for 29 CHCs in the two largest counties. The core model for MHIP was to include mental health care through the evidence-based CoCM (developed at the University of Washington), with CHPW providing funding for a behavioral health care manager who would be physically integrated into the CHC setting. The AIMS Center provided technical assistance and training for the program and worked with CHPW and the CHCs to ensure quality and adherence to the core components of the CoCM model.

In 2009, the program was expanded statewide and is currently in 100 CHCs and 30 community mental health centers, with continued support from the AIMS Center in training, technical assistance, and administration of a Web-based tracking system for the registries within the clinics (Unützer et al. 2012). The program continues to be funded by the state of Washington and is administered by CHPW in collaboration with Seattle and King County Public Health. The population for the pilot continues to include low-income adults who have temporary disability due to medical or behavioral health conditions and who are expected to be unemployed for at least 90 days (adults within the Disability Lifeline program). Others included in the population are veterans and their family members, the uninsured, low-income mothers and their children, and low-income older adults (Unützer et al. 2012).

MHIP outcomes point toward an effective model with reductions in inpatient medical admission, decreases in the number of arrests, changes in the way in which individuals used services (e.g., an increase in use of shelters and homeless services), and lower increases of homelessness (Association for Community Affiliated Plans 2014; SAMHSA-HRSA Center for Integrated Health Solutions 2014). However, their data suggested significant variation among the CHCs in quality and outcomes (Unützer et al. 2012). In an effort to improve the quality and standardization of the program as well as outcomes, the sponsors initiated a quality improvement program with a P4P incentive. Before the P4P, CHCs received full payment for the cost of the care managers; however, the P4P shifted this payment to 25% of the annual program funding, contingent on achievement of specific quality indicators (e.g., timely follow-up of patients, psychiatric consultation for those not improving, medication tracking, and other key components of the CoCM model) (Unützer et al. 2012).

The P4P incentive resulted in an increase in timely follow-up, the proportion of individuals who received a review by a psychiatrist, and the overall reduction in depression and depressive symptoms among patients served by these CHCs (Unützer et al. 2012). Even more interesting was that the time required for patients to reach a 50% or more reduction in depression and depressive symptoms decreased from 64 weeks to 25 weeks after implementation of P4P (Unützer et al. 2012), indicating that individuals were not only getting better at a higher rate, but they were getting better more quickly as a result of the CHC being incentivized to achieve quality outcomes through the provision of integrated care services.

This is one of the first examples of how P4P can improve behavioral health outcomes in a primary care setting. Although the cost savings data is still emerging and may take more time to materialize, MHIP demonstrates how many of the future models of finance will pair payment and quality and how incentives can ultimately lead to better care and more efficient care through more rapid improvement.

Rocky Mountain Health Plans: Colorado

Rocky Mountain Health Plans (RMHP) is an innovative health plan in Colorado, serving more than 200,000 members and nearly 190,000 other individuals through the Rocky Mountain Health Plans Foundation. In keeping with its commitment to physician-directed care and an emphasis on keeping members healthy, RMHP has aggressively sought to support the introduction of financially sustainable integrated care through its Medicaid Prime program. In 2012, the Colorado legislation passed House Bill 1281, requiring payment reform, including global payment reform pilots within the Accountable Care Collaborative program. RMHP used this opportunity for experimentation with payment to create Medicaid Prime.

Working with the University of Colorado Department of Family Medicine and the Collaborative Family Healthcare Association, RMHP has been testing a global payment budget for financially sustaining integrated behavioral health care in six practices in rural western Colorado. RMHP's Medicaid Prime program is unique in that it is not concerned with the model of clinical integration but rather is looking specifically at payment model sustainability. Specifically, the goals of Medicaid Prime are to determine if a global payment method will financially support and sustain behavioral health in primary care, understand how different payment models will affect clinical models of integration and their related costs, and test the real-world application of a global payment methodology on primary care practices that have integrated behavioral health. The lessons learned can then directly inform the state's policy, a central goal of the Colorado Department of Health Care Policy and Financing (Medicaid Department) and the Colorado legislature.

Under Medicaid Prime, practitioners are paid capitation for providing integrated care but also have the opportunity to access shared savings if the network's actual costs are lower than the projected trend or payments, with about 60% of the savings going to medical providers, 30% to BHPs, and 10% to RMHP. This capitation was determined from a cost-based budget, and the program sought to be very permissive regarding what was included in the budget, which amounted to a small incremental increase over the existing capitation. How providers use the global budget to integrate care is flexible, and integration is broadly defined. Wraparound supports and specialized services are all included, including visits that are not typically paid for through fee-for-service. Additionally, RMHP chose not to mandate provider credentials for the delivery of specific services, allowing for provider flexibility. Medicaid Prime also includes support for practitioners in estimating the incremental cost for integrating behavioral health and primary care in their practices by using an online tool created for this purpose.

While RMHP has had requirements about reporting activity to the health plan, they did not want to drive practitioners back to concentrating simply on activity level and so have sought to emphasize competency and outcomes over traditional licensure restrictions and service volume. Providers have benefited from having the flexibility to care for behavioral health needs without having to be concerned with how to configure that care in such a way as to create a billable service. As one RMHP executive said of using nontraditional interventions such as group care, which are not normally reimbursed in primary care, "What works can't be coded." This sentiment speaks to a major concern for providers engaged in integrated care across the county—many of the elements of effective integrated care are nonbillable (e.g., warm handoffs, curbside consultations, registry management). A health plan acknowledging this challenge and creating a path for provider-driven solutions in deciding elements of care is part of what makes this pilot so unique.

Although the study is ongoing, some lessons are already emerging. Unsurprisingly, it has been found that costs vary significantly with disparate personnel and integration activities, with lower costs for practices relying more on PCPs, medical assistants, and front office staff and higher costs associated with practices employing more licensed BHPs as well as extensive case and care management services. RMHP is convinced that to bring a more effective value-based payment model such as Medicaid Prime to scale, it will need to be multipayer, because without the participation of Medicaid and Medicare, a myriad of smaller pilots will not collectively result in a transformative reform of payment methods that incorporate consideration of the total cost of care.

Another central lesson from RMHP's Medicaid Prime program is that the administrative simplicity of Medicaid Prime has been an essential facet, not only with credentialing and provider requirements but also with network administration and plan benefits. And while some simplification efforts have resulted in cost savings, the move to capitated payment from fee-for-service has not only realized savings but has also been more conducive to team-based care because of the removal of coding as the primary revenue driver for providers. Challenges remain, as health plans and other entities still need data traditionally obtained through fee-for-service claims submission. Regulatory burdens that compromise efficiency also remain, but while paying capitation for comprehensive care may be increasingly common, Medicaid Prime is unique in its determination to give providers the necessary resources and freedom to provide integrated care, and then actively measuring the resulting impact on the total cost of care.

Coordinated Care Organizations: Oregon

Using patient-centered primary care homes, a model similar to the more familiar patient-centered medical homes, the Integrated Behavioral Health Alliance of Oregon (IBHAO) is defining the scope and standards of excellent, evidence-based behavioral health provision in the state of Oregon (for more information on Oregon's IBHAO and the definitions and minimum standards created for integrated behavioral health, see the CCO Oregon Web page: www.ccooregon.org/workgroups/IBHAO). This grassroots effort led by practitioners already engaged in integrated care has worked closely with payers, health systems, and the Oregon Health Authority to develop standards for integrated care and to codify important components into legislation, paving the way for Oregon's communities to integrate behavioral health and physical health services. Participation in the IBHAO is an all-volunteer effort by the providers involved, borne out of a commitment to developing a financially sustainable model for integrated care. Although there was some HRSA funding behind some of the early integrated care work in Oregon, financial support was preceded by a commitment to provide integrated care even if doing so resulted in a short-term financial drain.

Oregon's health care system uses local health entities called Coordinated Care Organizations (CCOs) to deliver health care and coverage for those enrolled in the state's Medicaid program. In contrast to many environments where payers span across the state or region and do not align with local coordinating entities, Oregon's Centers for Medicare and Medicaid Services (CMS) waiver allows money to trickle down through the CCOs to community-based providers. With the exception of the Eastern Oregon CCO, which spans across a large area because of its rural location, each CCO usually serves as payer and provider to no more than a few counties. Although they are all responsible for meeting 12 quality metrics for care provided within their locality, they are provided with a lot of flexibility on their approach. Therefore, the IBHAO had to fully engage the CCOs in statewide planning discussions and be flexible enough to allow for localized solutions. The IBHAO has focused their efforts in recent years on developing minimum requirements for "integration," standards that ultimately formed the basis for Senate Bill (SB) 832, which was signed into law in 2015 (for full text of the law, see https://olis.leg.state.or.us/liz/2015R1/Downloads/MeasureDocument/SB832/Enrolled). SB 832 is the beginning of bidirectional integration across the health system, increasing access to behavioral health care at the point where the patient presents. These standards, adapted from *A Guidebook of Professional Practices in Behavioral Health and Primary Care Integration* (Agency for Healthcare Research and Quality 2015), include seven domains, each with clear specifications regarding the requirements to meet that standard. The domains include access, comprehensiveness of services, integration of care teams, population-based focus, and use of psychiatric consultative services.

The IBHAO identified some key lessons that have come out of their experience thus far. The first was that the support of the Oregon Health Authority was crucial, even going so far as having a representative from the state in its workgroup. Another significant lesson was the importance of educating BHPs outside of primary care on how the efforts of the IBHAO were intended to complement rather than compete with their work, and how the financial support for IBHAO's work would ultimately be coming out of savings from elsewhere in the system rather than from behavioral health dollars. In order to maintain a strong primary care focus and have people actually doing the work in primary care to set the standards, the IBHAO was limited to BHPs (e.g., psychologists, social workers, licensed therapists) working in primary care and did not include BHPs working in traditional specialty behavioral outpatient care. However, at the time leading up to SB 832, Oregon's BHPs were also engaged in their own integration efforts apart from the CCO Oregon structure and were operating in parallel, but not in conjunction with, the work of the IBHAO. Although these different viewpoints were ultimately compromised in legislation, this challenge could have been avoided had these groups emphasized coordination of their work earlier. More broadly, they recognized a need to create buy-in across multiple levels as they advocated for a new approach to financing integrated care.

What Do These Case Studies Tell Us?

These four case studies provide real-life stories about how integration was designed in a health care system, received funding, and proceeded to demonstrate positive outcomes. The case studies also illustrate the ongoing challenges that exist in blending medical and behavioral health policy, finance, and ultimately delivery. What is important in these large-scale pilots, although different in the specific components of the model, is that they point toward important improvements in the quality of care for the populations served as well as meaningful cost savings. As noted in the section "Reimbursement-Related Policy Barriers" earlier in this chapter, one of the challenges to integration is ensuring that the provider (i.e., practices doing integration) also receives the financial benefit and that there is not purely a financial savings at the population or payer level. Examples such as MHIP highlight how both goals can be met while also tying financial success to improved health—a genuine success for the Triple Aim of improved health outcomes, improved patient experience, and lower costs (Berwick et al. 2008). The future will hold more iterations of these models mirroring the balance between achievement of cost savings at a population level with payment incentives for the practices choosing to implement integration.

RECENT GAME CHANGERS— PAYING FOR EVIDENCE-BASED INTEGRATION

Health care policy makers, payers, and providers are increasingly focused on quality improvement and accountability, using evidence-based practices as the vehicle to provide care that is effective and efficient, as demonstrated by models like DIAMOND, MHIP, and RMHP. Increasingly, more payment is being connected to specific evidence-based programs. In recent years, the CoCM has been recognized as an evidence-based integrated care practice by SAMHSA and as a best practice by the Surgeon General's report on mental health (Unützer et al. 2013; U.S. Department of Health and Human Services 1999). Although there are a number of other practice-tested methods currently being used to treat behavioral health conditions within primary care settings, many of these variations do not incorporate all of the essential features of CoCM and thus are not considered an evidence-based practice (Unützer 2015). This distinction is important, as many of those interviewed for this chapter noted the paramount importance of engaging payers in conversations about the evidence behind their selected practice. For example, the DIAMOND Steering Committee included Minnesota Medicaid's major payers from the outset so that they could engage in discussions related to the strong evidence base of CoCM before the initiative's launch.

As further recognition of the evidence for the CoCM, CMS has made two recent changes that offer additional financial support for its use. The first was a change to the Medicare Physician Fee Schedule (and CPT code 99490), which provides PCPs additional payments for chronic care coordination and telehealth services. It is the provision of reimbursement for non-face-to-face encounters that has been an important shift for providers. Many of the core CoCM functions done by the behavioral care manager were previously non-billable activities, such as telephonic follow-up or care coordination. The code provides support for non-face-to-face encounters and includes reimbursement for addressing depression and anxiety (AIMS Center, https://aims.uw.edu/cms-finalizes-rule-cover-collaborative-care). The code also opens the provider requirements so that a physician is not required to do these activities, which instead can be done by care managers and BHPs. Covered activities include the development of a care plan, the monitoring of symptoms and outcomes, medication reconciliation, reviewing self-management goals, and caseload consultation, with the key being that these services can now be reimbursed without face-to-face contact (for more information, see CMS guidance for eligibility and other elements at www.cms.gov/Outreach-and-Education/Medicare-Learning-Network-MLN/MLNProducts/Downloads/ChronicCareManagement.pdf). Adequate support of care management functions has been a central barrier to integration, and this code created a new avenue for payment. However, there has been limited use of this code in collaborative care settings because of the complicated provisions for services and documentation.

Going even further, CMS has announced that effective January 2017 there are three new CPT codes for supporting the CoCM. Use of these codes will require providers to demonstrate that they are meeting the core principles and effective components of implementation of the CoCM (see Chapter 1, "Elements of Effective Design and Implementation"). These new CPT codes provide a whole new level of support for many of the key elements of the CoCM model (patient engagement, brief interventions, psychiatric consultation, regular caseload review of the registry, and repeat measurement of progress toward goals; see Table 8–1). Once a month, the PCP will bill these codes for the core (traditionally nonbillable) tasks, while continuing to allow traditional psychotherapy codes to be billed in addition if that service is also provided. As described in the section "Reimbursement-Related Policy Barriers" earlier in this chapter, the lack of reimbursement for these core tasks has prohibited investment in integration and, specifically, the evidence-based CoCM, and these new CPT codes offer welcome relief.

Additionally, in December 2016, the U.S. Department of Health and Human Services announced the selection of eight states to participate in the Section 223 Certified Community Behavioral Health Clinic (CCBHC) demonstration project. The CCBHC initiative represents a federally driven push toward a behavioral health accountable care reimbursement model by establishing standardized certification criteria for community behavioral health clinics, promoting the integration of behavioral health with physical health care, and reimbursing CCBHCs through an FQHC-like prospective payment system (PPS) (Substance Abuse and Mental Health Services Administration 2015). The selected states, which comprise Minnesota, Missouri, Nevada, New Jersey, New York, Oklahoma, Oregon, and Pennsylvania, begin to implement their 2-year demonstration programs between January 1 and June 30, 2017 (U.S. Department of Health and Human Services 2016). Each of the selected states participated in the CCBHC planning year, during which they developed one of two types of PPSs designed to work within the scope of their state Medicaid plans. The PPS options from which the states selected are the following (Substance Abuse and Mental Health Services Administration 2015):

1. A cost-based, per clinic rate that is paid through a fixed, *daily* rate for all CCBHC services provided to a Medicaid beneficiary, with an *optional* Quality Bonus Payment (QBP) for achieving a variety of CMS- and state-specified measures[1] (see footnote next page); or

2. A cost-based, per clinic rate that is paid through a fixed, *monthly* rate for all CCBHC services provided to a Medicaid beneficiary. With this option, the monthly rate varies according to clients' clinical conditions, and states have flexibility to decide exactly how PPS rates will vary based on their local needs. In addition, states who choose this option are *required* to make a QBP to CCBHCs who achieve the CMS- and state-specified measures.[1]

Each state calculated its selected PPS to reimburse certified sites for all CCBHC services, including many that relate to integrated care (e.g., conducting primary care screening and monitoring of health risk for selected chronic conditions, leading interdisciplinary care teams in partnership with primary care partners). Of the eight states who were selected to implement demonstration projects, six have chosen to implement daily PPS rates, with all but one of those states opting to also include QBPs, while the other two chose a monthly PPS rate and QBPs. Regardless of whether providers are operating within a CCBHC demonstration state, this initiative represents a move toward payment models that promote greater flexibility and accountability for integrated care provision, and the CCBHC model can be used as a framework for BHPs interested in working with their state legislature, payers, and primary care partners to enhance their ability to provide integrated care.

FUTURE MODELS

Changes in CMS reimbursement and numerous policy changes such as Medicare reform (Medicare Access and Children's Health Insurance Plan Reauthorization Act, Merit-Based Incentive Payment System, and Alternative Payment Models), as well as models such as MHIP, point toward the future of value-based payment models. These new models will drive financing and quality with a focus on specific and measurable outcomes. There is significant evidence that integrated care not only improves patient satisfaction and health outcomes but is a cost-efficient mechanism to accomplish these aims. Yet it is also clear that in a system where such savings do not necessarily accrue to those who are making the investment in integrated care, market

---

[1]The CMS-specified QBP measures are primarily derived from the Medicaid Adult and Child Core Set measures. For a complete listing of the federally mandated CCBHC QBP measures, see Appendix III—Section 223 Demonstration Programs to Improve Community Mental Health Services Prospective Payment System (PPS) Guidance (Substance Abuse and Mental Health Services Administration 2015, pp. 9–10).

TABLE 8–1. Centers for Medicare and Medicaid Services temporary
G-codes for the Collaborative Care Model (CoCM)

Codes specific to the CoCM

G0502: Initial psychiatric collaborative care management, first 70 minutes
in the first calendar month of behavioral health care manager activities, in
consultation with a psychiatric consultant, and directed by the treating
physician or other qualified health care professional, with the following
required elements:

- Outreach to and engagement in treatment of a patient directed by the
  treating physician or other qualified health care professional

- Initial assessment of the patient, including administration of validated
  rating scales, with the development of an individualized treatment plan

- Review by the psychiatric consultant with modifications of the plan if
  recommended

- Entering patient in a registry and tracking patient follow-up and
  progress with the registry, with appropriate documentation, and
  participation in weekly caseload consultation with the psychiatric
  consultant

- Provision of brief interventions by using evidence-based techniques,
  such as behavioral activation, motivational interviewing, and other
  focused treatment strategies

G0503: Subsequent psychiatric collaborative care management, first
60 minutes in a subsequent month of behavioral health care manager
activities, in consultation with a psychiatric consultant, and directed by
the treating physician or other qualified health care professional, with
the following required elements:

- Tracking patient follow-up and progress with the registry, with
  appropriate documentation

- Participation in weekly caseload consultation with the psychiatric
  consultant

- Ongoing collaboration with and coordination of the patient's mental
  health care with the treating physician or other qualified health care
  professional and any other treating mental health providers

- Additional review of progress and recommendations for changes in
  treatment, as indicated, including medications, based on
  recommendations provided by the psychiatric consultant

TABLE 8–1. Centers for Medicare and Medicaid Services temporary G-codes for the Collaborative Care Model (CoCM) *(continued)*

- Provision of brief interventions by using evidence-based techniques such as behavioral activation, motivational interviewing, and other focused treatment strategies

- Monitoring of patient outcomes by using validated rating scales and relapse prevention planning with patients as they achieve remission of symptoms and/or other treatment goals and are prepared for discharge from active treatment

G0504: Initial or subsequent psychiatric collaborative care management, each additional 30 minutes in a calendar month of behavioral health care manager activities, in consultation with a psychiatric consultant, and directed by the treating physician or other qualified health care professional (list separately in addition to code for primary procedure) (Use G0504 in conjunction with G0502 or G0503)

Behavioral health integration code not specific to the CoCM

G0507: Care management services for behavioral health conditions, at least 20 minutes of clinical staff time, directed by a physician or other qualified health care professional time, per calendar month (for other models of integration)

Note. For a Healthcare Common Procedure Coding System (HCPCS) Medicare payment summary and related information, see University of Washington AIMS Center: Cheat Sheet on CMS Final Rule for 2017 Medicare Payments for Integrated Behavioral Health Services. February 15, 2017. Available at: https://aims.uw.edu/sites/default/files/CMS_FinalRule_2017_CheatSheet.pdf.

---

forces alone will not encourage the necessary transformation to bring widespread implementation of integrated care into the larger health care system. Fortunately, examples abound of creative efforts to develop such alignment, just a few of which were highlighted in this chapter. Approximately $26–$48 billion in annual savings for commercial insurers, Medicare, and Medicaid could be realized from implementing effective integrated care (Melek et al. 2014). Multiple other studies cited in this chapter point to positive and significant return on investments, and evidence will continue to mount for the wisdom in enacting further payment reform that will support more integrated approaches.

But this evidence needs to drive action and reform, building on the work already being done by innovative state and federal policy makers, progressive integrated health systems, and pioneering practitioners. Although value-based payment models and other reimbursement models that more closely align payment with outcomes and value are rapidly proliferating, a very large proportion of health care dollars are still spent via traditional volume-based mechanisms. If and when a tipping point is reached, evidence-based integrated care should be, by definition, financially sustainable. Until that time, significant efforts must remain in place to support innovation, offset start-up and ongoing nonreimbursable costs, and break down policy barriers that contribute to misaligned incentives and "business as usual."

REFERENCES

Agency for Healthcare Research and Quality: A Guidebook of Professional Practices for Behavioral Health and Primary Care Integration: Observations from Exemplary Sites (AHRQ Publ No 14-0070-1-EF). Rockville, MD, Agency for Healthcare Research and Quality, March 2015. Availabe at: https://integrationacademy.ahrq.gov/sites/default/files/AHRQ_AcademyGuidebook.pdf. Accessed March 2, 2017.

Association for Community Affiliated Plans: SAMHSA-HRSA Center for Integrated Health Solutions Safety Net Health Plans: Working with providers in underserved areas to integrate behavioral health and primary care. 2014. Available at: http://communityplans.net/portals/0/fact%20sheets/ACAP%20CIHS%20Physical%20Behavioral%20Health%20Integration.pdf. Accessed September 23, 2016.

Berwick DM, Nolan TW, Whittington J: The triple aim: care, health, and cost. Health Aff (Millwood) 27(3):759–769, 2008 18474969

Brown B, Crapo J: The key to transitioning from fee-for-service to value-based reimbursement. Salt Lake City, UT, HealthCatalyst, 2014. Available at: https://www.healthcatalyst.com/wp-content/uploads/2014/08/The-Key-to-Transitioning-from-Fee-for-Service.pdf.

California Primary Care Association: Integrated behavioral health care: an effective and affordable model. 2007. Available at: http://www.cpca.org/cpca/assets/file/policy-and-advocacy/active-policy-issues/mhsa/integrationbrief.pdf. Accessed September 23, 2016.

California Primary Care Association: The California alternative payment methodology pilot. 2014. Available at: http://www.cpca.org/cpca2013/assets/File/Policy-and-Advocacy/Active-Policy-Issues/Payment-Reform/2014–12–10-CPCA-CA-APM-RealSmartReform.pdf. Accessed September 23, 2016.

Colorado Health Foundation: The Colorado blueprint for promoting integrated care sustainability. March 2012. Available at: http://www.integration.samhsa.gov/TCHF_IntegratedCareReport.pdf. Accessed September 23, 2016.

Gracey D: Health care providers and value based reimbursement, Health Management Associates. 2015. Available at: https://www.healthmanagement.com/wp-content/uploads/Health-Care-Providers-and-Value-Based-Reimbursement.pdf. Accessed September 23, 2016.

Harris J: Approaches to behavioral health integration: integration through innovation. MassHealth, 2013. Available at: http://www.mass.gov/anf/docs/hpc/hpc-mh-bh-integration-final-04-02-13.pdf. Accessed September 23, 2016.

Hostetler C, Sisulak L, Cottrell E, et al: Origins in Oregon: The alternative payment methodology project. Health Affairs, 2014. Available at: http://healthaffairs.org/blog/2014/04/14/origins-in-oregon-the-alternative-payment-methodology-project. Accessed September 23, 2016.

Houy M, Bailit M: Barriers to behavioral and physical health integration in Massachusetts. 2015. Available at: http://bluecrossfoundation.org/sites/default/files/download/publication/Barriers%20to%20Behavioral%20and%20Physical%20Health%20Integration%20in%20MA_Final.pdf. Accessed September 23, 2016.

Institute for Clinical Systems Improvement: The DIAMOND program: treatment for patients with depression in primary care. 2014. Available at: https://www.icsi.org/_asset/rs2qfi/DIAMONDWP0614.pdf. Accessed September 23, 2016.

Katon W, Unützer J, Fan MY, et al: Cost-effectiveness and net benefit of enhanced treatment of depression for older adults with diabetes and depression. Diabetes Care 29(2):265–270, 2006 16443871

Klein S, Hostetter M: In focus: Integrating behavioral health and primary care. New York, The Commonwealth Fund, August/September 2014. Available at: http://www.commonwealthfund.org/publications/newsletters/quality-matters/2014/august-september/in-focus. Accessed September 23, 2016.

Melek SP, Norris DT, Paulus J: Economic impact of integrated medical-behavioral health care. Milliman, Inc., 2014. Available at: https://www.psychiatry.org/File%20Library/Psychiatrists/Practice/Professional-Topics/Integrated-Care/Milliman-Report-Economic-Impact-Integrated-Implications-Psychiatry.pdf. Accessed September 23, 2016.

Mountainview Consulting Group: Integrating primary care and behavioral health services. Bureau of Primary Health Care: Managed Care Technical Assistance Program. 2016. Available at: https://www.apa.org/practice/programs/rural/integrating-primary-behavioral.pdf. Accessed September 23, 2016.

Nardone M, Snyder S, Paradise J: Integrating physical and behavioral health care: promising Medicaid models. The Kaiser Commission on Medicaid and the Uninsured, 2014. Available at: http://kff.org/report-section/integrating-physical-and-behavioral-health-care-promising-medicaid-models-issue-brief. Accessed September 23, 2016.

New York State Department of Health: A path toward value based payment: New York state roadmap for Medicaid payment reform. 2015. Available at: https://www.health.ny.gov/health_care/medicaid/redesign/dsrip/docs/vbp_roadmap_final.pdf. Accessed September 23, 2016.

Pietruszewski P: A new direction in depression treatment in Minnesota: DIAMOND program, Institute for Clinical Systems Improvement, Bloomington, Minnesota. Psychiatr Serv 61(10):1042–1044, 2010 20889647

Physicians for a National Health Program: Single payer system cost? 2016. Available at: http://www.pnhp.org/facts/single-payer-system-cost. Accessed September 23, 2016.

Rafeyan R: Outcomes and cost effectiveness of collaborative care disease management approach in depression patients. 2012. Available at: http://www.namcp.org/journals/jmcm/articles/15–1/Depression.pdf. Accessed September 23, 2016.

Rovner J: Debate sharpens over single-payer health care, but what is it exactly? National Public Radio, 2016. Available at: http://www.npr.org/sections/health-shots/2016/01/22/463976098/debate-sharpens-over-single-payer-health-care-but-what-is-it-exactly. Accessed September 23, 2016.

SAMHSA-HRSA Center for Integrated Health Solutions: How to Integrate Primary Care into a Behavioral Health Setting: Lessons Learned from the SAMHSA Primary and Behavioral Health Care Integration Program (presentation). September 26, 2014. Available at: http://www.integration.samhsa.gov/about-us/Integrating_Behavioral_Health_and_Primary_Care_Webinar_9-26-14_.pdf. Accessed September 23, 2016.

Substance Abuse and Mental Health Services Administration: Planning Grants for Certified Community Behavioral Health Clinics. 2015. Available at: https://www.samhsa.gov/sites/default/files/grants/pdf/sm-16-001.pdf. Accessed February 23, 2017.

Sunflower Foundation: Integrated care. 2015. Available at: http://www.sunflower-foundation.org/what_we_do/health_care/integrated_care. Accessed September 23, 2016.

University of New Mexico: Integrated addiction and psychiatry. 2015. Available at: http://echo.unm.edu/nm-teleecho-clinics/integrated-addiction-and-psychiatry-clinic. Accessed September 23, 2016.

University of Washington AIMS Center: Collaborative care. 2015. Available at: https://aims.uw.edu/collaborative-care. Accessed September 23, 2016.

Unützer J: Proposed CMS revisions to payment policies published in 7/15/2015 Federal Registry: comments on collaborative care models for beneficiaries with common behavioral health conditions. 2015. Available at: https://aims.uw.edu/sites/default/files/AIMS_CMS_Comments.pdf. Accessed September 23, 2016.

Unützer J, Katon WJ, Fan MY, et al: Long-term cost effects of collaborative care for late-life depression. Am J Manag Care 14(2):95–100, 2008 18269305

Unützer J, Chan YF, Hafer E, et al: Quality improvement with pay-for-performance incentives in integrated behavioral health care. Am J Public Health 102(6):e41–e45, 2012 22515849

Unützer J, Harbin H, Schoenbaum M, et al: The collaborative care model: an approach for integrating physical and mental health care in Medicaid Health Homes. 2013. Available at: https://www.medicaid.gov/State-Resource-Center/Medicaid-State-Technical-Assistance/Health-Homes-Technical-Assistance/Downloads/HH-IRC-Collaborative-5–13.pdf. Accessed September 23, 2016.

U.S. Department of Health and Human Services: Mental Health: A Report of the Surgeon General. Rockville, MD, U.S. Department of Health and Human Services, Substance Abuse and Mental Health Services Administration, Center for Mental Health Services, National Institutes of Health, National Institute of Mental Health, 1999

U.S. Department of Health and Human Services: HHS selects eight states for new demonstration program to improve access to high quality behavioral health services. December 21, 2016. Available at: https://www.hhs.gov/about/news/2016/12/21/hhs-selects-eight-states-new-demonstration-program-improve-access-high-quality-behavioral-health. Accessed February 23, 2017.

Waldman B, Dyer MB, Waldinger J: Implementing state payment reform strategies at Federally Qualified Health Centers. Robert Wood Johnson Foundation. 2015. Available at: http://www.bailit-health.com/articles/2015-1215-bhp-rwjf-implementing-state-payment-reform-strategies.pdf. Accessed September 23, 2016.

Washington State Health Care Authority: Federally Qualified Health Centers provider guide. 2016. Available at: http://www.hca.wa.gov/assets/billers-and-providers/fqhc_bi_01012016-03312016.pdf. Accessed March 2, 2017.

APPENDIX 8–A

Performance Grid Example

The following grid provides an illustration of how to examine payment issues. It outlines an example of how an organization may start to map the billing and coding potential by payer and for each provider or team member on the integrated team. Although the grid example has only one provider (for a social worker), this grid would be used for all providers in the clinic—for mapping out which codes are billable under each payer for each type of clinician and team member.

The authors thank Virna Little for the permission to share this resource. The table has been adapted from an Excel document for the purposes of this text.

Licensed Master Social Worker

Payers	90791	90832	90834	90837	90853	96150	96151	99366	99367	99368	98967	98968
Medicaid												
Medicare												
1199												
ADAP												
Aetna												
Affinity												
AmidaCare												
CenterLight												
CDPHP												
Cigna												
Elderplan												
Empire BCBS/HealthPlus												
Empire BCBS (HMP/PPO)												
Fidelis												
GHI												
HealthFirst												
HIP												
MagnaCare												
MetroPlus												
MVP												
MultiPlan												

Note. ADAP = AIDS Drug Assistance Program; BCBS = Blue Cross Blue Shield; CDPHP = Capital District Physicians' Health Plan; GHI = Group Health Incorporated; HIP = Health Insurance Plan; HMP/PPO = Health Maintenance Organization/Preferred Provider Organization; MVP = MVP Health Care.

Performance and Outcome Measures for Integrated Care

A great deal of research supports the Collaborative Care Model (CoCM), and the evaluation of key components of efficacy has provided several reliable constructs on which to build a performance program. There is an inherent logic in the idea of "treating the whole person," of attaching the head to the body, and creating a seamless connection between physical and behavioral health. But that logic must be validated through measurement and data in order for programs to demonstrate outcomes and be accountable for the care provided. As an emerging innovation, evaluation also provides information on core components of integrated care and which factors lead to desired impacts and which are less vital. Determining which program components "matter" is essential to the long-term sustainability of the approach and ensures that effort (time and resources) in development of integrated care programs has a return on investment, both in patient outcomes and in cost containment.

At the clinical practice level, demonstration of outcomes is increasingly important. With policy and clinical emphasis on patient-centered care, there is greater accountability of patient improvement and patient expectation (see Chapter 7, "Policy and Regulatory Environment"). The same drivers are raising expectations for primary care settings to engage in population health and thereby increase accountability with a broader impact. Policy changes and payers are also placing an emphasis on performance and increasingly connecting payment to outcomes (see Chapter 8, "Financing Integrated Care"). As the emphasis on value-based payment or pay-for-performance intensifies, there is even more importance for interventions that have documented effectiveness and can demonstrate that the defined impact can be replicated through consistent and reliable implementation.

Although primary care providers (PCPs) are typically attentive to quality of care, recent decades of increasing demands, changes to reimbursement structures, and an emphasis on efficiency (not always quality) have meant that the metric of focus has been productivity (e.g., how many patients are seen in a day). A shift back to value and quality is both empowering and welcome but no less challenging. Establishing accountability and demonstrating outcomes in a busy primary care practice that is in a changing reimbursement environment requires another set of procedural changes and more broadly a culture shift. Although providers care about quality, they have not always welcomed accountability to outcomes (especially if the outcomes are determined by external stakeholders such as payers). If we hope to merge these important themes in the pursuit of the Triple Aim (i.e., better outcomes, reduced cost of care, better patient experience of care), then all levels of the system must embrace and become passionate advocates for evaluation- and measurement-based care.

Integrated care programs need to incorporate evaluation from the start by laying the foundation of program assessment (fidelity to what is demonstrated to be effective) and patient and population outcomes in order to support sustainability. These elements of assessment need to inform the individual providers on change in practice and success in measurement-based treating to target and inform the patient in reaching desired goals. At the same time, these metrics need to be able to demonstrate patient improvement, population improvement, and ultimately value to the payers and system at large. At the most basic level, evaluation of integrated care comes down to these two central questions: **1) Are we doing what we said we were going to do?** and **2) Are patients benefiting from our approach to care?**

Clearly, the first question sets the stage for the second; practice teams need to demonstrate a shift in the practice of care by changing practice (*process metrics*) in order to lead to a change in clinical performance (*outcome metrics*). The shift in practice with integrated care includes having the tools and workflow in place to efficiently screen, measure, and review data to inform measurement-based decision making. When systems of care try to shift to integration and measure patient outcomes without these process metrics assessing accountability to the effective components of models, they set providers and patients up for failure on the outcome side. Finally, choosing measures that already exist in the flow and are regularly documented in the medical record help support the care team by providing the data points their quality team uses to measure outcomes. Adding additional forms and tools must be carefully considered. They can be used with specific populations or limited periods of time in order to not overload an already busy workforce. Just shadowing an actual patient's flow through the practice from check-in at the front desk, exam room visit, and pharmacy stop to clinic exit helps the practice stay focused on the primary aim of improving patient care.

PROCESS MEASURES

Examples of collaborative care process outcomes include the rate of screening completed and timely rescreening, the number of warm handoffs occurring between medical providers and behavioral health providers (BHPs), whether the huddle is occurring on time and has all team members present, inclusion of patient goals in care planning, whether routine review of registry is occurring, and others specific to the team and population. Groups may also include a team effectiveness or team functioning measure such as TeamSTEPPS (see the Agency for Healthcare Research and Quality Web page: www.ahrq.gov/teamstepps/index.html) or the Team Climate Inventory (Bosch et al. 2008). Additional process metrics are outlined in Table 1.

An example of process measures being incorporated into pay-for-performance models comes from the Mental Health Integration Program (MHIP) in Washington (see Chapter 8, "Financing Integrated Care"). Three of the five quality measures required are focused on the frequency of contact between the behavioral health staff and the patient. Measuring frequency of patient contact, frequency of PCP and BHP patient handoffs, number of and type of patient encounters on the same date, and provider productivity all give a picture of the access patients have to behavioral health services in primary care and demonstrate that a practice is incorporating core elements of collaborative care. Determining the percentage of patients who receive a screening or diagnostic interview, or who have a documented care plan, also establishes program fidelity and effective components. MHIP is an example of a payment model that has explicitly tied process components and evidence-based program components to improved clinical outcomes.

TABLE 1. Sample process measures and metrics

Outcome measure broadly defined	Example measure	Example metric	Reference or standard
Patient identification	Depression screening (recommend universal use of the PHQ-9, self-scored by patient)	% of patients screened with PHQ-2 or PHQ-9	NQF 712; U.S. Preventive Services Task Force 2013; Healthcare Effectiveness Data and Information Set (National Committee for Quality Assurance 2017)
		% of patients with positive PHQ-2 (score >2) who completed the PHQ-9	—
		% of patients with positive PHQ-9 (score >9)	—
		% of patients with positive PHQ-9 score diagnosed with major depression or persistent depressive disorder	—
		Further division of PHQ-9 scores by % of patients with mild (score 5–9), moderate (score 10–15), moderately severe (score 16–20), and severe (score 20–27) depression	—

TABLE 1. Sample process measures and metrics *(continued)*

Outcome measure broadly defined	Example measure	Example metric	Reference or standard
Patient identification *(continued)*	Alcohol screening	% of patients with AUDIT-C screening	NQF 1661
		% of patients with positive AUDIT-C score (men >3, women >2)	—
		% of patients with positive AUDIT-C score given the full AUDIT	—
		% of patients with positive AUDIT score who received a documented brief intervention	NQF 2152
	Anxiety	% of adults and children screened for anxiety	—
		% of patients with positive GAD-7 (score >9)	—
		% of patients with positive GAD-7 score with a diagnosis of an anxiety disorder	—
Engagement and follow-up	Engagement and best practice follow-up	% of patients with ≥1 follow-up contact with the care manager or BHP within 4 weeks of initial contact	Bao et al. 2016; Mental Health Integration Program 2012 *Suggested benchmark:* 50%

TABLE 1.   Sample process measures and metrics *(continued)*

Outcome measure broadly defined	Example measure	Example metric	Reference or standard
Measurement-based treat to target	Ongoing symptom monitoring at each contact	% of patients with ≥1 measure based on valid instruments (PHQ-9) recorded at each follow-up	Mental Health Integration Program 2012
	Registry review	% of patients not improving (<5-point decrease in PHQ-9) who received a documented psychiatric consultation between weeks 8 and 12	Bao et al. 2016; Mental Health Integration Program 2012 *Suggested benchmark:* 80%
Ongoing engagement	Tracking contact	No periods of ≥60 days between enrollment and discharge when no contact occurs	Mental Health Integration Program 2012
Patient-centered care	Inclusion of patients in treatment planning	% of care plans with patient goals identified	National Quality Strategy Priority 2 (U.S. Department of Health and Human Services 2016a)
	Patient activation	% of patients with improved activation measured by tools such as the Patient Activation Measure (PAM)	PAM (Insignia Health 2017); Hibbard et al. 2004

TABLE 1.   Sample process measures and metrics *(continued)*

Outcome measure broadly defined	Example measure	Example metric	Reference or standard
Team process			
	Huddle consistency	Number of team members by discipline at daily huddle	—
	Collaboration	% of patients who received both PCP and BHP contact on same day, to measure internal collaboration	—
	Multidisciplinary team meetings	Number of team meetings in a 6-month period	—
		Number of team meetings and attendance of team members by discipline	—
	Team culture	Use of validated team measures such as the Team Climate Inventory	Bosch et al. 2008

Note.   — = reference or standard not available; AUDIT = Alcohol Use Disorders Identification Test; AUDIT-C = Alcohol Use Disorders Identification Test—Consumption; BHP = behavioral health provider; GAD-7 = Generalized Anxiety Disorder 7-Item Questionnaire; NQF = National Quality Forum; PCP = primary care provider; PHQ-2 = Patient Health Questionnaire–2; PHQ-9 = Patient Health Questionnaire–9.

OUTCOME MEASURES

As the example from the MHIP in Washington highlights (see Chapter 8, "Financing Integrated Care"), the process components are the foundation for the patient outcomes, which represent the second question for the evaluation process: Do patient's health outcomes improve? This question has been a long-term challenge for behavioral health practice. Measuring physical health improvement has a long history of measurement with proven and now standard practice metrics, such as the hemoglobin A_{1c} for diabetes. Vital signs are other examples of a core set of physical health metrics. In the CoCM and other forms of integrated care, a central practice change is using universal screening to more objectively capture individual risk for mental health and substance use disorders. Although these metrics are based on patient report, they have been demonstrated to adequately measure emotional distress and mood. Screening tools provide excellent, reliable, initial, and ongoing assessment of a patient's level of symptomatology, but follow-up with an interview by a PCP or a BHP is essential to determine the actual diagnosis. The use of validated screening tools is a shift in practice that balances subjective clinical assessment with research-based assessment tools to evaluate patient improvement. As the MHIP example highlights, the goal is to identify more accurately individuals who are not responding to care so that interventions can be "stepped up" (see Chapter 1, "Elements of Effective Design and Implementation") in intensity to reach improvement.

Following screening and confirmation of diagnosis there is a need to reliably provide a mechanism for ongoing measurement of symptoms, with tools such as the Patient Health Questionnaire–9 (PHQ-9) or the Generalized Anxiety Disorder 7-Item Questionnaire (GAD-7). Although these tools are not perfect, they have provided reliable estimates of response to treatment in many clinical studies and have been widely and successfully used to track progress.

As value-based payment is incorporated into practice, there will be an intensified effort to identify the right set of measures that demonstrate effectiveness and individual and population improvement. At this juncture, clinical practice outcomes could include a combination of measured medical improvements (e.g., hemoglobin A_{1c}, blood pressure, and body mass index) with reduction in symptoms of depression, anxiety, and substance use. Other measures of patient outcomes assess patient improvement through evaluation of use and need for higher levels of care (e.g., reduction in emergency department use, reduction in readmission to inpatient care—both psychiatric and medical—reduction in pharmacy use, improved follow-up with primary care scheduled visits, and reduction in referral to psychiatry), demonstrating the assumption that as individuals improve, their use of higher-level services decreases. Other correlated patient improvement outcome measures include a reduction of missed days at work, stable pain medication management, or successful completion of a patient care plan. Table 2 outlines a sample of these measures and corresponding metrics.

The traditional approach to measuring patient improvement is identifying a patient population, describing a specific intervention, and seeing if that intervention makes a difference. This traditional approach to research and validation is essential to continuing to establish integrated care as a valuable and logical approach to patient care. Evaluation for providers who are caring for a wide range of patients, from newborns to elders, with both physical and behavioral health problems on a wide continuum of problem severity, is particularly important as findings can highlight successful real-world solutions. Provider partnerships with research institutions and payers are needed to support direct service assessment that can answer whether or not integrated care indeed meets the Triple Aim in health care. The refrain that effective care requires a team for clinical integration implementation is just as true for evaluation.

This appendix is a beginning to a discussion about the role of evaluation and quality improvement in integrated care. By no means is it a comprehensive discussion or listing of measures for organizations and providers to consider. Instead, the goal is to outline the importance of measurement-based practice, an evaluation of the model that will need to demonstrate the role of both process and outcome measures. These can be linked to measurement of broader outcomes, such as patient and provider satisfaction, improved population health, and value-based savings that can support reimbursement and sustainability of the approach.

TABLE 2.   Sample outcome measures and metrics

Outcome measure broadly defined	Example measure	Example metric	Reference or standard
Patient improvement	Depression response to treatment	% of patients diagnosed with depression or dysthymia with an initial PHQ-9 score >9, who had ≥50% reduction in their PHQ-9 score at 6 and 12 months	NQF 1884 and 1885 *Suggested benchmark:* >40%
	Depression remission	% of patients diagnosed with depression and an initial PHQ-9 score >9 who had remission (PHQ-9 score <5) at 6 months and 12 months	NQF 711 and 710 *Suggested benchmark:* >20%
	Multiple chronic conditions	% of patients with 2 or more chronic conditions and depression that had improvement in hemoglobin A_{1c} (HbA_{1c}) levels and PHQ-9 score	Katon et al. 2010
	Anxiety response to treatment	% of patients with GAD-7 score >9 with 50% reduction in symptoms	—
	Anxiety remission	% of patients with GAD-7 score <5	Spitzer et al. 2006

TABLE 2. Sample outcome measures and metrics *(continued)*

Outcome measure broadly defined	Example measure	Example metric	Reference or standard
Patient improvement *(continued)*	Alcohol use: risky drinking	% of patients over the past month with a positive AUDIT score (> 7 for women and > 8 for men) who had reduction in alcohol use to low-risk drinking levels, defined as • ≤14 drinks/week for men under age 65; ≤7 drinks/week for women under age 65 • ≤7 drinks/week for men and women over age 64	U.S. Department of Health and Human Services 2016b
	Alcohol use: heavy drinking	% of patients with a positive AUDIT score who over the past month had a reduction in number of days of heavy drinking (≥5 drinks at one time in men and ≥4 drinks at one time in women) % with a positive AUDIT who stopped drinking (abstinence)	U.S. Department of Health and Human Services 2016b
	Attention-deficit disorder/ hyperactivity disorder (ADHD)	% of patients with a positive score on the Vanderbilt Assessment Scale diagnosed with ADHD who had a reduction in the total score of items 1–18	—

TABLE 2. Sample outcome measures and metrics *(continued)*

Outcome measure broadly defined	Example measure	Example metric	Reference or standard
Patient improvement *(continued)*	Adolescent depression	% of adolescents diagnosed with depression or dysthymia, with an initial PHQ-A score >9, who had ≥50% reduction in their PHQ-A score at 6 and 12 months	Standard for performance not currently available but is most comparable to adult standard (see "Depression response to treatment" at beginning of table)
	Adolescent functioning	% of patients with Pediatric Symptom Checklist score >14 who had a decrease in symptoms	NQF 0722
Utilization measures	Reduction of frequent emergency department use	% reduction in number of patients with frequent emergency department visits (defined as >4 visits in the past year)	Centers for Medicare and Medicaid Services 2014
	30-day readmission to inpatient (psychiatric and medical) care	% reduction in number of patients with a 30-day readmission to an inpatient service	Centers for Medicare and Medicaid Services 2016
	Specialty behavioral health utilization	% decrease in referrals to specialty behavioral health services	—

TABLE 2. Sample outcome measures and metrics *(continued)*

Outcome measure broadly defined	Example measure	Example metric	Reference or standard
Cost of care	Reduction in total overall health care costs	% reduction in the total overall health care costs	Unützer et al. 2008
Satisfaction with integrated care	Patient-perceived health status	% of patients with increase in healthy days on the Centers for Disease Control Health-Related Quality of Life	Centers for Disease Control and Prevention 2016
	Patient satisfaction	% of patients with improved satisfaction on satisfaction measures	Wen and Schulman 2014
	Provider satisfaction	% of providers with improved satisfaction in work experience	Levine et al. 2005
	Retention of providers	Number of providers who leave practice in a 6- or 12-month period	—
Physical care of serious mental illness (SMI)[a]	Tobacco use screening and follow-up for people with SMI or alcohol or other drug dependence	% of patients age 18 years and older with an SMI or alcohol or other drug dependence who received a screening for tobacco use, with follow-up for those identified as a current tobacco user	NQF 2600

TABLE 2. Sample outcome measures and metrics *(continued)*

Outcome measure broadly defined	Example measure	Example metric	Reference or standard
Physical care of SMI[a] *(continued)*	BMI screening and follow-up for patients with SMI	% of patients age 18 years and older with an SMI who received a screening for BMI and follow-up for those who were identified as obese (BMI ≥ 30 kg/m²)	NQF 2601
	Controlling high blood pressure for patients with SMI	% of patients age 18–85 years with SMI who had a diagnosis of hypertension and whose blood pressure was adequately controlled during the measurement year	NQF 2602
	Diabetes care for patients with SMI: HbA_{1c} testing	% of patients age 18–75 years with SMI and diabetes (type 1 and type 2) who had HbA_{1c} testing during the measurement year	NQF 2603
	Diabetes care for patients with SMI: HbA_{1c} control (<8.0%)	% of patients age 18–75 years with SMI and diabetes (type 1 and type 2) whose most recent HbA_{1c} level during the measurement year is <8.0%.	NQF 2608

[a]See discussion of reverse or bidirectional integration in Chapter 5, "The Primary Care Provider."

Note. —=reference or standard not available; AUDIT=Alcohol Use Disorders Identification Test; BMI=body mass index; GAD-7=Generalized Anxiety Disorder 7-Item Questionnaire; NQF=National Quality Forum; PHQ-A=PHQ-9 modified for adolescents; PHQ-9=Patient Health Questionnaire—9.

REFERENCES

Bao Y, Druss BG, Jung HY, et al: Unpacking collaborative care for depression: examining two essential tasks for implementation. Psychiatr Serv 67(4):418–424, 2016 26567934

Bosch M, Dijkstra R, Wensing M, et al: Organizational culture, team climate and diabetes care in small office-based practices. BMC Health Serv Res 8(180), 2008 18173837

Centers for Disease Control and Prevention: Health-related quality of life. 2016. Available at: https://www.cdc.gov/hrqol. Accessed September 23, 2016.

Centers for Medicare and Medicaid Services: Reducing Nonurgent Use of Emergency Departments and Improving Appropriate Care in Appropriate Settings. January 16, 2014. Available at: https://www.medicaid.gov/Federal-Policy-Guidance/Downloads/CIB-01-16-14.pdf. Accessed February 16, 2017.

Centers for Medicare and Medicaid Services: Readmissions Reduction Program (HRRP). April 18, 2016. Available at: https://www.cms.gov/medicare/medicare-fee-for-service-payment/acuteinpatientpps/readmissions-reduction-program.html. Accessed February 16, 2017.

Gardner W, Murphy JM, Childs G, et al: The PSC-17: a brief pediatric symptom checklist including psychosocial problem subscales: a report from PROS and ASPN. Ambulatory Child Health 5:225–236, 1999

Guo T, Xiang YT, Xiao L, et al: Measurement-based care versus standard care for major depression: a randomized controlled trial with blind raters. Am J Psychiatry 172(10):1004–1013, 2015 26315978

Hibbard JH, Stockard J, Mahoney ER, Tusler M: Development of the Patient Activation Measure (PAM): conceptualizing and measuring conceptualizing and measuring activation in patients and consumers. Health Serv Res 39(4 Pt 1):1005–1026, 2004 15230939

Insignia Health: Patient Activation Measure, 2017. Available at: http://www.insignia health.com/products/pam-survey. Accessed February 16, 2017.

Katon WJ, Lin EH, Von Korff M, et al: Collaborative care for patients with depression and chronic illnesses. N Eng J Med 363(27):2611–2620, 2010 21190455

Levine S, Unützer J, Yip JY, et al: Physicians' satisfaction with a collaborative disease management program for late-life depression in primary care. Gen Hosp Psychiatry 27(6):383–391, 2005 16271652

Mental Health Integration Program: Five 2012 quality aims. 2012. http://aims.uw.edu/sites/default/files/QualityAimsExample.pdf. Accessed September 23, 2016.

National Committee for Quality Assurance: HEDIS & Performance Measurement. Available at: http://www.ncqa.org/hedis-quality-measurement. Accessed February 22, 2017.

Spitzer RL, Kroenke K, Williams JB, Löwe B: A brief measure for assessing generalized anxiety disorder: the GAD-7. Arch Intern Med 166(10):1092–1097, 2006 16717171

Substance Abuse and Mental Health Services Administration: National Behavioral Health Quality Framework. October 30, 2014. Available at: http://www.samhsa.gov/data/national-behavioral-health-quality-framework. Accessed September 23, 2016.

Unützer J, Katon WJ, Fan MY, et al: Long-term cost effects of collaborative care for late-life depression. Am J Manag Care 14(2):95–100, 2008 18269305

U.S. Department of Health and Human Services: National Quality Strategy: Overview. March 2016a. Available at: https://www.ahrq.gov/workingforquality/nqs/overview.htm#s22. Accessed February 16, 2017

U.S. Department of Health and Human Services: Rethinking Drinking: Alcohol and Your Health, p 4. NIH Publ No 15-3770. May 2016b. Available at: https://pubs.niaaa.nih.gov/publications/RethinkingDrinking/Rethinking_Drinking.pdf. Accessed February 16, 2017.

U.S. Preventive Services Task Force: Final recommendation statement: alcohol misuse: screening and behavioral counseling in primary care. May 2013. Available at: http://www.uspreventiveservicestaskforce.org/Page/Document/Recommendation StatementFinal/alcohol-misuse-screening-and-behavioral-counseling-interventions-in-primary-care. Accessed September 23, 2016.

Wen J, Schulman KA: Can team-based care improve patient satisfaction? A systematic review of randomized controlled trials. PLoS One 9(7):e100603, 2014

Index

Page numbers printed in **boldface** *type refer to tables or figures.*

CPSIA information can be obtained
at www.ICGtesting.com
Printed in the USA
BVHW090026230922
647541BV00006B/13